Can a Health Care
Market Be Moral?

Can a Health Care Market Be Moral?

A Catholic Vision

Mary J. McDonough

Georgetown University Press/Washington, D.C.

As of January 1, 2007, 13-digit ISBN numbers have replaced the 10-digit system.

13-digit	10-digit
Paperback: 978-1-58901-157-1	Paperback: 1-58901-157-0

Georgetown University Press, Washington, D.C.

Library of Congress Cataloging-in-Publication Data

McDonough, Mary J.
  Can a health care market be moral : a Catholic vision / Mary McDonough.
    p. ; cm.
  Includes bibliographical references and index.
  ISBN-13: 978-1-58901-157-1 (pbk. : alk. paper)
  ISBN-10: 1-58901-157-0 (pbk. : alk. paper)
  1. Medical ethics—Religious aspects—Catholic Church. 2. Medicine—Religious aspects—Catholic Church. 3. Medical economics—Religious aspects—Catholic Church. I. Title.
  [DNLM: 1. Health Care Sector—ethics—United States. 2. Catholicism—United States. 3. Social Justice—United States. W 74 AA1 M478c 2007]
  R725.56.M334 2007
  174.2—dc22

2006031182

♾ This book is printed on acid-free paper meeting the requirements of the American National Standard for Permanence in Paper for Printed Library Materials.

14 13 12 11 10 09 08 07   9 8 7 6 5 4 3 2
First printing

Printed in the United States of America

For my father, James B. McDonough

CONTENTS

ACKNOWLEDGMENTS

First of all, I would like to thank Owen Cummings and Abbot Peter Eberle of Mount Angel Seminary. I had the privilege of studying theology under these two fine men, who live out their faith every day in their lives.

This book began as a dissertation for my PhD at Graduate Theological University in Berkeley, California. I wish to thank my dissertation readers, Michael Mendiola and Al Jonsen, who provided me with their keen insights into my project. Also, my brother, Jim McDonough, and a friend, Dr. Debbie Erdman, who served as much-needed proofreaders for the original text.

Finally, there are two men to whom I owe so much. Rich Gula, who served as my adviser for five years at GTU and as chair of my dissertation committee, spent many thankless hours editing my work. He was a source of constant encouragement throughout the process. And this project never would have come into being without Daniel Callahan. Dan gave me the inspiration and confidence to write a book. I had the privilege of serving as his research assistant for a brief time. During this wonderful experience I was able to use the library and research staff at the Hastings Center and spend time with Dan, learning how to write a book and how to think like a writer. Dan helped me refine my ideas and provided me with an abundance of encouragement and enthusiasm. I simply would not have been able to write this book without his continual help and support. I am forever grateful to both of these inspirational men.

INTRODUCTION

There is an old joke that goes like this: "How many University of Chicago economists does it take to change a light bulb?" The answer: "None, because the market will take care of it." The joke continues: "How many political scientists does it take to change a light bulb?" The answer: "None, because the government will take of it!" So goes the ongoing ideological debate. Who is better qualified to oversee a national economy: the market, with its invisible hand, or government, with its intrusive regulations? Many economists, politicians, and public policymakers have fallen into the trap of virtually advocating either the market alone or maximum involvement of government.

The Roman Catholic Church has fallen into a similar snare. Although the Church recognizes some value of a market economy and abhors Marxism and communism, it views laissez-faire capitalism with suspicion. With the market system's emphasis on individualism and self-interest, the Church sees it as failing to uphold tenets the Church teaches as being primary: the dignity of each human being and the pursuit of the common good. The *Catechism of the Catholic Church* (1994) states that the Church has "refused to accept, in the practice of 'capitalism,' individualism and the absolute primacy of the law of the marketplace over human labor.... Regulating [the economy] solely by the law of the marketplace fails social justice, for 'there are many human needs which cannot be satisfied by the market.'"[1] Rather than relying on the human self-interest as expressed by the market, the Church looks toward government to serve the common good by regulating and overseeing the various institutions and associations that make up society, thereby ensuring that the principles of justice are upheld.

But what about the funding and distribution of health care? Today the health care system in the United States is a mire of rapidly increasing costs and continually declining numbers of insured. Efforts to achieve universal health care coverage have chronically failed. Yet health care costs are rapidly rising. In 1970, 7.6 percent of the nation's gross domestic product (GDP) was spent on health care. By 2004 that figure had risen to 15 percent, the highest in the world.[2] Moreover, in 2003 insurance premiums rose 13.9 percent, greatly outpacing the 2.2 percent annual inflation rate.[3] That was the third consecutive year of double-digit premium increases and represented the greatest increase since 1990.[4] The number of uninsured people is growing as well. In 2004 approximately 44.5 million people in the United States were uninsured.[5] There is general agreement on why affordable, fair distribution of health care is growing increasingly difficult: the rising number of elderly people as a significant proportion of the population, the impact of new technologies and the intensified use of older ones, and an increasing public demand for ever better health care. Yet there is no consensus on what approach to distributing health care will best address this situation.

This book addresses the morality of using market mechanisms to provide for the funding and distribution of health care. Countries throughout the world, even countries with long-established government-run universal health care systems, are increasingly turning over parts of their health care systems to private entities or using other market mechanisms to control skyrocketing costs. With increasing pressures to contain costs, the market may seem to be the only feasible alternative. In the United States in part because of the Bush administration, the market issue is becoming more and more important on the national scene.

The Catholic health care system is the largest private nonprofit provider of health care in the United States. Catholic health care represents a major voice in the ongoing debate on health care reform. Traditionally, the Catholic Church has understood access to health care as fundamental to the common good. With the papacy of John XXIII (1958–63), Catholic justice theory moved from a teleological language of goals to the deontological language of human rights, whereby the human person is not the mere subject of economic and social life but, rather, is the purpose of it. As John XXIII wrote in *Pacem in terris (Peace on Earth)*, the common good is actually defined by a notion of dignity that encompasses certain rights: "Any human society, if it is to be well-ordered and productive, must lay down as a foundation this principle, namely, that every human being is a person. . . . Precisely because he is a person he has rights and obligations flowing directly . . . from his very nature. And these rights and obligations are universal and inviolable."[6] These include the right to food, shelter, employment, political participation, *and* medical care.[7] The right to health care is also developed in the U.S. Bishops' 1981 "Pastoral Letter on Health and Health Care": "Every person has a basic right to adequate health care. . . . Access to that health care which is necessary and suitable for the proper development and maintenance of life must be provided for all people, regardless of economic, social or legal status."[8]

However, the Catholic Church has never explicitly stated how such a right is to be guaranteed. There has been almost no effort within Catholic theological circles to grapple with the details of how to fund and distribute health care. Although the Catholic Health Association of the United States has set forth guidelines for health care reform, these represent only broad generalizations about the financing of health care and rely heavily on government for implementation and oversight. The market has been treated by Catholic theology as a black or white choice, a yes or a no. That picture does not reflect the wide range of market practices, many of them within universal health care systems and aiming to improve, not undermine, those systems.

There is a large amount of Catholic literature on rather broad notions of justice and health care, but it is difficult to find any literature dealing with the details of market practices or the thinking of leading health care economists. The purpose of this book is to fill in a gap in Catholic social thought by assessing the use of market ideas and practices in the provision of health care. This discussion presents a nuanced evaluation of the market in light of recent debates among secular health care economists, showing when the use of market practices would and would not be consistent with Catholic social teaching, making recommendations about the possibilities, and limits, of market practices in health care, and presenting a Catholic vision of health care.

The driving theological question is not whether the market or government should be in charge of the financing and distribution of health care. Rather, the question is whether some market practices are compatible with Catholic social thought and may be used to control health care costs. Organizational details and efficiency are important, but health care is not solely about economic issues. There are several deep, underlying value premises that I will analyze—such as the ways in which health, life, suffering, and death are interpreted—that affect how health care is perceived and delivered.

Justice and the Catholic Church

I will explore the development of Catholic social justice theory to draw out implicit convictions, which I will then use to assess two different approaches to health care. In determining which market practices are compatible with Catholic social thought, a range of issues need to be addressed. First is the concept of justice. The Catholic Church has a rich social justice tradition. From Saint Augustine (354–430) to the present, Catholic justice theory has evolved dramatically. Yet certain themes dominate Catholic social thought. The dignity of the human person, a recognition of the social interdependence of humans, the promotion of the common good, a special obligation to the poor and vulnerable, and an obligation of stewardship over the world's resources—essential themes in Catholic social justice theory—are used to evaluate whether a political, social, or economic institution or system is just. Further, the Gospel itself demands justice in the world. And it is the Church's responsibility, according to a 1971 statement by the Synod of Bishops, "to proclaim justice on the social, national, and international level, and to denounce instances of injustice, when the fundamental rights of man and his very salvation demand it."[9]

Moreover, Catholic social thought provides unique ways of understanding the world and avenues of meaning. Through a Christian interpretive framework, Catholic thought brings unique interpretations to many values underlying the human condition. For example, health care cannot be assessed apart from certain convictions about human dignity, the purpose of life and death, and the problem of suffering. The notion of justice and the unique Christian framework found within Catholic social thought are not simple, but they are essential to understanding whether a health care market is moral.

Capitalism, Health Care, and Catholic Social Thought

With an understanding of the foundational Catholic themes of justice, we then approach the topic of the market, which is complex. Historian Jerry Muller provides a basic definition of the concept as "the systematic exchange of labor and the products of labor" within a capitalistic system.[10] Catholic social thought has frequently judged capitalism and its market mechanisms as failing the principles of social justice. The Church is involved in economic matters because it believes that economic systems affect all in society. Economic systems should not help merely a few people or even a majority of people. Rather, according to Catholic thought, they must promote the common good of all people. Several modern papal documents, beginning with the labor encyclical of Leo XIII (papacy 1878–1903), issued in 1891, call into question the morality of the market system. Furthermore, because of its view that government is better at promoting the common good, Catholic social thought generally prefers it over private entities when it comes to managing political, social, and economic institutions.

For centuries the Catholic Church has also involved itself in medical issues through moral theology and pastoral medicine. The early Christian church viewed medicine as a vocation of healing inspired by Christ himself. Between the seventh and twelfth centuries, lay doctors were quite rare, and most of medicine was practiced behind the walls of monasteries. Although medicine is no longer dominated by people in religious orders, the Catholic Church continues to have a large presence in health care. It is, in fact, one of the major voices calling for universal health care coverage. Still, with the abundance of expensive medical technology available as well as public demand for better and better health, increasing inequities in access to care, and severe cost-containment problems, Catholic health care, along with all health care systems, is struggling to stay afloat in the muddy waters of the provision of health care. Can Catholic social thought overcome its suspicion of the market in order to help finance a universal health care system? My aim is to look at this question and offer some solutions on how this can be done.

Economic Theory, Market Mechanisms, and Health Care

Although the definition of the market and Catholic social thought's critique of it may appear simple, they are more complex when applied to the world of health care. The provision of health care is a morass of funding, organizational, and distribution mechanisms. There is a multitude of different kinds of health care services. This section will review the various types of market mechanisms commonly used in health care and assess their advantages and disadvantages. Not only are the mechanisms themselves important, but health outcomes among the various types of health care systems are critical for discerning the morality of a health care market. Hence, I will look at health care data from several nations and assess health outcomes.

Health care economic theory is another important piece of the health care puzzle that is essential to address. I will provide a summary of the debate among health care economists. The critical issue here is whether the market should be used at all to fund and organize health care. Health care economists do not agree; some argue that health care is so unique that market mechanisms are doomed to fail. Others contend that relying on the market is the only way health care systems can survive.

Even if certain market mechanisms are used for health care funding, though, who will oversee the organization and distribution of health care? On the one hand, some argue that government, with its seemingly unending rules, regulations, and red tape, is completely unable to accomplish such a task. On the other hand, others in the health care field argue that in view of the growing numbers of uninsured and evidence of poor health outcomes for the uninsured, government, on the federal and more-local levels, is the only entity capable of guaranteeing equitable access to health care.

Two Approaches to Health Care

The complexities of the market system and unique characteristics of health care are not the sole issues involved in this debate. There are two major approaches to health care that require our attention: the market organization approach and the value dimension approach. The *market organization approach* is exemplified in the works of four secular thinkers: Milton Friedman, Regina Herzlinger, Mark Pauly, and Alain Enthoven. The market organization approach emphasizes profit, private enterprise, and competition. Incentives promote cost effectiveness, and legal contracts are used to establish relationships between insurers and the insured, between insurers and providers, and often between purchasers and providers. This approach promotes for-profit institutions as health care providers and emphasizes a system where, although some federal and state regulations exist, most of the decisions about insurance products and the distribution of health care are made by private actors.[11] One of the primary goals of this approach is to address how market practices can produce a more efficient system than government can.

I choose those four figures because, though they all basically take the market organization approach, they represent the spectrum in the debate. Milton Friedman, the famed Nobel laureate, epitomizes the market ideology point of view. His love of the market is not merely founded on an appreciation of market economic theory, but flows from an underlying ideology based on a broader political agenda, reflecting an intense dislike of government and an emphasis on individual freedom and democracy. His perspective has a large and powerful following, including conservative publications such as the *Wall Street Journal* and the *Economist*, as well as politicians such as George W. Bush. Friedman argues that the problems plaguing the health care system can be cured through the privatization of medical care, requiring the elimination of most third-party payments and the use of major medical catastrophic insurance.

Regina Herzlinger, a professor at the Harvard Business School, has been deeply influenced by the thought of Friedman. She advocates the two Cs and one *I*: individual *choice*, consumer *control*, and *information* to enable more control and better choices within the health care system. She views health care as yet another consumer market to be mastered. In fact, she prefers to call people using the health care system "consumers" instead of "patients." Although Herzlinger, like Friedman, is a market zealot, she acknowledges that government should have some role in the provision of health care by subsidizing insurance policies for the poor and others who are vulnerable in society.

A third advocate of the market organization approach to health care is Mark Pauly. A professor at the University of Pennsylvania's Wharton School, Pauly has his own plan for health care, called Responsible National Health Insurance. This calls for several complex tax credits and subsidies to ensure universal coverage. He allows for a small role for government, through subsidization of insurance policies. Pauly argues that the use of the market will result in efficiency and choice, which will in turn keep health care costs in check.

The final market advocate I examine is Alain Enthoven, who advocates managed competition. He believes that an unregulated free market will not work. As an alternative, he invokes microeconomic principles. His plan calls for sponsors to act on behalf of subscribers to structure and adjust the market to guarantee that insurance coverage can be bought by everyone. Government would be responsible for several functions, such as enacting laws requiring everyone to have insurance coverage, determining the minimum level of acceptable insurance benefits, designating fallback plans for people who do not get coverage in the private market, and subsidizing a risk pool for people in the high-risk category.

The second approach to health care that I will examine is the *value dimension approach*. Its foremost advocate is Daniel Callahan, who calls for a reconsideration of the basic goals of medicine, particularly the notion of medical progress. His interest is not merely on how to organize and manage health care but on the underlying value premises that drive our health care systems. Callahan believes that we can contain health care costs more easily if we change our unlimited desire to live better and longer lives at all costs, a desire that continues to drive the market organization approach. Callahan faults the market approach for its failure to define finite goals and for its favoring individual desire and choice. As an alternative, Callahan advances an approach that is grounded in the meaning of health, in appropriate medical goals, and in economic sustainability.

In this book I will examine these two approaches to health care distribution in light of Catholic social thought. I will assess their implicit convictions regarding social responsibility and the dignity of the person, as these pertain to distributing health care, in light of Catholic social teaching. In doing so, I will turn to the Magisterium and natural law ethicists, such as Richard McCormick and Charles E. Curran, who have written specifically on the contribution of Catholic social teaching to health care reform.

Catholic Values and Health Care

Implicit in Catholic social thought is universal health care. But is universal health care consistent with market principles? I argue that it is—but only under the following circumstances. First, certain underlying values influencing health care must be redefined. Second, the cost pressure problem must also be reconceptualized as involving two main variables: system efficiency and organization, and the ends and goals of medicine. Catholic social thought, with its standard of justice and Christian framework of meaning, will help in this redefining and reconceptualizing. I will review the Catholic literature on certain underlying values that affect the human condition, such as the meaning of life, health, and death, as well as literature on the goals of medicine and the rationing of medicine as they pertain to the cost control problem. I will show how Catholic social thought can accept certain market mechanisms for the funding and distribution of health care, provided these mechanisms are integrated with the value dimension approach espoused by Callahan and interpreted within a Christian framework of meaning.

Plan of the Book

I begin in chapter 1 with a broad survey of the justice tradition in Catholic social thought. Here I draw out and define six central themes that characterize justice: the dignity of the human person, a recognition of the social interdependence of humankind, the promotion of the common good, a special obligation to the poor and vulnerable, a unique notion of stewardship over the world's resources, and a Christian interpretive framework of meaning. These themes will guide the subsequent analysis of political, economic, and social institutions.

Following that chapter I look at Catholic social thought on capitalism and health care. I begin with a brief overview of the history of capitalism in order to clarify the term and set the stage for the debate. Then I examine the Catholic

Church's response to capitalism in light of the major tenets of Catholic social thought on economics. I also review the Church's specific critique of capitalism in modern papal documents and the U.S. bishops' pastoral letter on economics. To show the diversity of Catholic opinions on capitalism, I examine the opposing positions of American conservative Michael Novak and Catholic liberation theology. The first part of chapter 2 closes with some conclusions about Catholic social thought, justice, and capitalism.

The second part of chapter 2 deals with Catholic social thought on health care. I review the Church's involvement in health issues and then examine the Catholic Health Association's document on health care reform and the U.S. Catholic bishops' pastoral letter on health care in order to understand why the Church even involves itself in health care.

Chapter 3 deals with health care economic theory and specific market mechanisms devised to finance health care. Here I review the major economic arguments for and against the use of the market in health care. Then I identify and discuss the advantages and disadvantages of the most commonly used market mechanisms within an international context. I also classify several nations according to their uses of market mechanisms in health care, in order to make broad comparisons of the health outcomes of different health systems.

Chapter 4 explores market organization approaches to health care by examining the proposals of Milton Friedman, Regina Herzlinger, Mark Pauly, and Alain Enthoven. Chapter 5 examines the work of Daniel Callahan and his value dimension approach to health care. I use Catholic social thought to assess each of these approaches.

The book concludes with a chapter that develops a Catholic vision of health care. Here I draw upon Catholic social teaching to show that a Catholic vision of health care can accept some market mechanisms to curb costs—but only when used along with certain elements of the value dimension approach promulgated by Daniel Callahan.

I began this journey as an adamant supporter of government-run, universal health care, the kind of system found in Canada. I had no idea how complicated the funding and distribution of health care really is. While working on this book, I have come to appreciate the market system a bit more. I recognize that it can contribute both to the funding of health care as well as to the organization of the system so that it is better managed and more effective. Still, working on this book also reinforced my belief that all people should have access to basic health care. The present health care system in the United States is a travesty. The statistics on poor health outcomes, missed opportunities, and financial ruin that frequently occur among the uninsured or underinsured is staggering.

For a health care market to be moral, our health care system must undergo fundamental changes both in the way in which health care is organized and the way in which we perceive certain underlying values regarding the human condition. These changes will not be easy. They will require major reversals in thinking by the health care "consumer," the medical profession, and the pharmaceutical industry, among other interested parties. But without these changes, the U.S. health care system will continue to serve fewer and fewer people and cost more and more.

Notes

1. United States Catholic Conference, *Catechism of the Catholic Church*, no. 2425.
2. Callahan and Wasunna, *Medicine and the Market*, 228.
3. Kaiser Family Foundation, "Employee Health Benefits: 2003 Annual Survey," 13.
4. Ibid.
5. Kaiser Commission, *Health Care in America, 2004 Data Update*, 10.
6. John XXIII, *Pacem in terris*, no. 9, 132.
7. Ibid., nos. 11–27.
8. National Conference of Catholic Bishops, "U.S. Bishops' Pastoral Letter," 402.
9. Synod of Bishops, 1971, "Justice in the World," 294.
10. Muller, *Mind and the Market*, xvii.
11. Peterson, "Introduction: Health Care," 12.

Justice in Catholic Social Thought

What is justice? The meaning of this abstract term has been disputed for centuries by secular and Catholic philosophers from before ancient Greece to today. The great philosopher Plato thought justice meant a commonwealth where "each one must practice one of the functions in the city, that for which his nature made him naturally most fit."[1] For Aristotle justice is the virtue preeminently concerned with right relationships with others.[2]

John Locke linked justice to property rights: "The great and chief end therefore, of men's uniting into commonwealths, and putting themselves under government, is the preservation of their property."[3] On the other hand, Karl Marx expressed justice like so: "From each according to his ability, to each according to his need."[4] Among contemporary political philosophers, Robert Nozick sees justice in terms of property rights: The allocation of scarce resources is not so much the question of distributive justice as is the manner by which a holding is acquired.[5] John Rawls presents a very different case, contending that justice is based on principles of equal liberty and opportunity for all.[6]

The Catholic Church has a rich justice tradition. Rooted in its social teachings, Catholic justice theory has evolved dramatically over hundreds of years. Beginning with Saints Augustine and Thomas Aquinas, who provide an essential foundation for Catholic justice theory, to the more recent encyclicals of John Paul II, Catholic justice theory is continually being reinterpreted and applied to contemporary situations.

Augustine and Aquinas

Augustine's main contribution to Catholic social thought is found in his political teachings. Key to his notions about civil society is his teaching on virtue.

Augustine sees humans as social beings who have a unique ability to form relationships and build political communities. This idea is critical to Catholic social thought. To Augustine, people choose to live in political society, and more importantly, only through living in society can people become fully human.

Augustine argues that not only do people flourish by living in a political society, but it is the virtue of justice that directs all citizens to the common good of the city (society). Without justice, there can be no true commonwealth at all. Much of Augustine's thought on justice is found in his *City of God*, a book written in response to the barbarian Goth invasion of Rome in AD 410. Many Roman pagans blamed Rome's defeat on the influence of Christianity. They believed that by abandoning the pagan gods, Rome had become weak and susceptible to attack.

Against this background Augustine was asked to refute the charge that Christianity was responsible for Rome's decline. To make his argument in Book 2 of *City of God* (the entire work is divided into parts and further divided into "books"), Augustine analyzes the elements needed to create a republic. He looks to Cicero, who, before the birth of Christ, stated that a true commonwealth cannot exist without justice.[7] Augustine describes the absence of justice as a condition whereby "there is no longer the welfare of the people . . . bound together by a common recognition of rights, and a mutual cooperation for the common good."[8] Augustine defines the common good as a "common pursuit" that unites humankind.[9] In Book 19, using Cicero's definition of a true commonwealth again, Augustine questions whether Rome was ever a true commonwealth. He concludes that it was not, because Rome never possessed "a mutual recognition of rights and a mutual co-operation for the common good."[10] With his notion of the common good, Augustine lays the cornerstone in the foundation of Catholic social thought.

Augustine also gives the concept of justice a Christian perspective: Justice is giving God what is due Him, and the common good is the unification of a people bound by their faith in and love of God.[11] Augustine concludes that the only commonwealth that embodies true justice is the City of God, where all is rightly ordered toward a love of God and neighbor, for just people "love God as He should be loved and one's neighbor as oneself."[12] Hence, Augustine links justice, the common good, and Christianity.

The great Scholastic thinker Thomas Aquinas (1224–74) believed that Aristotelian philosophy was very compatible with Christianity, and he therefore reinterpreted Aristotle in light of Christian revelation. Aquinas grounds his theology in the Aristotelian view of human nature: People have a communitarian nature, whereby what is good for each person is connected to the good of the community.[13] Whereas Augustine thought that a truly just society could exist only in the City of God, yet to be achieved, Aquinas lived at a time when Christianity dominated all walks of life in Western Europe. This included political life. Aquinas argues that since the family cannot provide humans with everything they need to sustain life, political society is necessary. Humans therefore must belong to a political society to achieve full humanity.[14] People do not give up their individual freedom to live in a political society, nor is the state viewed as coercive. Rather, it is through the political community that people perfect their humanity. This conviction that social relationships allow humankind to flourish helps refine the notion of the common good. People cannot become virtuous or just on their own. Rather, this occurs through and within the community. Moreover, the whole of the community is more important than the specific interest of an individual member.

In further keeping with the thought of Aristotle, Aquinas teaches that virtues are habits that orient people toward perfection. Unlike Aristotle, however, for whom human perfection is defined as *eudaimonia*, or excellence, Aquinas believes human perfection is beatitude, or union with God.

The virtue of justice dominates Aquinas's social, economic, and political thought because it is essential in guiding human action toward the common good. Aquinas defines justice in the classic sense as "to pay what is due,"[15] but it has a special importance among the virtues because it has both the character of a general virtue as well as the character of an individual virtue. *General*, or *legal, justice* is a general virtue in that it directs all the acts of the virtues toward the common good.[16] *Particular justice* regulates the dealings of one individual in relation to another. It is a social norm that guides people in their actions with one another. Finally, there are two species of justice. *Distributive justice* governs relationships between the whole community, or state, and smaller groups. It is primarily concerned with the allotment or distribution of public goods. *Commutative justice* regulates dealings between individuals, such as contractual agreements.[17]

Another major contribution Aquinas makes to Catholic social thought is his concept of law. He suggests that there are four different kinds of law. The *eternal law* is God's wisdom, which comes from God and is the source of all creation. It directs the world toward its fulfillment.[18] *Divine law* is the part of eternal law revealed by God to humankind, such as the Decalogue and the Great Commandment. Divine law is necessary so people can know what God wants them to do or to avoid. *Human law*, or *positive law*, governs public life and promotes the common good.[19] Finally, Aquinas recognizes *natural law*. A difficult concept to define, natural law is an extrabiblical source of moral knowledge, yet it is another way people participate in the eternal law. Natural law allows for people to use their reason to attempt to understand and evaluate what is ethical behavior. Though natural law is carried out through human reason,[20] this is not human reason in the narrow sense of the term; rather, by understanding their purpose and meaning, people can participate more fully in God's plan for the world.

The Influence of *Rerum novarum*

Modern Catholic teaching about justice began with Pope Leo XIII's *Rerum novarum* (*On the Condition of Labor*). Although there had been social teaching emanating from the Vatican prior to Leo XIII's encyclical, his pontificate (1878–1903) marks the beginning of presenting an official body of systematic authoritative social teaching in encyclicals, papal letters to the bishops. Published in 1891, *Rerum novarum* addresses several particularly relevant issues. Prior to this encyclical, the Church had resisted issuing stances on contemporary social and political issues. However, the social, economic, and political changes in nineteenth-century Western Europe, brought on by industrialization, scientific advancements, and nationalism, had rattled the Catholic Church and begged for attention.

The year 1848 was a time of political upheaval in Europe. In February, Karl Marx and Friedrich Engels published one of the most influential documents of socialism and of the century, the *Communist Manifesto*. Revolutions occurred later that year in both Berlin and Vienna. This was also a time of anticlericalism and nationalism in much of Europe. In 1870 the Papal States were lost. The Church could not avoid the reality of the secularization of much of Catholic Europe.[21]

The world was changing economically, as well. The industrial revolution left an immense mark on Western Europe, whose economies shifted from agrarian based to industrial and urban based. This change not only caused an upheaval in social systems but contributed to increased unemployment rates and housing shortages in urban centers. The dominance of factories within the new industrial system created serious concerns over working conditions and the frequent use of child labor. Workdays were often very long, and the wages were extremely low. Employees were often required to work on Sundays. Many factories were unsanitary, and most manufacturers did not provide any type of care for disabled workers.

During this time the Catholic Socialism movement began. Social Catholics were concerned about the social and economic upheavals caused by the industrial revolution. Their views consisted of a combination of progressive and traditional positions. Some Social Catholics proposed a corporative model of society, wherein people would be organized according to vocational groups including both workers and employers. Known as corporatism, this movement attempted to revive the guilds of the Middle Ages in the belief that the unification of workers and employers would allow the two groups to share common ground.[22] In hope of bringing about economic harmony, corporatism tried to represent a compromise between the intense individualism of capitalism and the encompassing collectivism of socialism.

In an attempt to address some of these volatile political, economic, and social issues, Pope Leo XIII wrote *Rerum novarum*. The encyclical contains several key elements that have been extremely influential in Catholic justice theory. The foremost of these is Leo XIII's emphasis on the inherent dignity of the human person. Certainly, Leo XIII was not the first to subscribe to the importance of human dignity. After all, the concept's Christian roots are biblical. The theology of human dignity is derived from the conviction that humankind is created in the image of God (Gen 1:26–27). Human dignity enshrines the capacities for reason and free will, the indispensable aspects of the moral dimension of being a person. Human dignity cannot be removed from someone nor renounced by anyone endowed with it. Moreover, human dignity is confirmed not only by our being created *imago Dei* but also by the covenant created between God and the people of Israel, which reflected God's powerful love and devotion not only to Israel but to the whole of humankind. The New Testament affirms human dignity through the incarnation, death, and resurrection of Jesus, for "God so loved the world that He sent His only son" (Jn 3:16).[23]

Still, the significance of human dignity was often ignored until Leo XIII's papacy. For many years the Catholic Church often rejected the world's approach toward human rights. For example, Pope Pius VI (papacy 1775–99) criticized the French Revolution's *Declaration of the Rights of Man* in 1790 because it was seen as promoting secular notions of individual freedoms, such as freedom of religion and freedom of conscience.[24] This antagonism toward secular concepts of rights continued into the nineteenth century.[25]

Leo XIII changed all of this with his encyclical. Toward the beginning of *Rerum novarum*, he writes his famous statement "Man is older than the State."[26]

In other words, the dignity of the person is the measure by which all political, legal, and social institutions are to be judged. People are never merely instruments of the political or social order. Rather, they are the primary focus of these institutions. Therefore, the purpose of political and social institutions is to serve the person.

Early on in his encyclical, Leo XIII expressly rejects socialism and equates the right to property to the right of families to self-preservation.[27] He argues that families need private property to ensure that they have food and other basic requirements needed for survival.[28] He sees the socialist state as usurping these rights and concludes that "the main tenet of socialism, the community of goods, must be utterly rejected."[29]

Yet, government is not excluded from serving its citizens. On the contrary, respecting human dignity requires that government help the people. It has a duty to act in accordance with the common good: "Whenever the general interest of any particular class suffers, or is threatened with, evils which can in no other way be met, the public authority must step in to meet them."[30]

Finally, Leo XIII brings together the concept of human dignity and a theory of social institutions.[31] Using the concept of commutative justice, he argues that workers have certain duties, such as to do labor agreed upon, not to injure property, and never to riot. Workers also have specific rights, including the right to a just wage, the freedom to enter into wage contracts, and the right to organize unions. These rights require the ability to enter freely into private agreements, an obligation to uphold such agreements, and a requirement that they be fair.[32]

Moreover, the role of social relationships is key to Leo XIII's understanding of justice. The good of the community, rather than the good of particular individuals, should be the ultimate goal of its members: "All citizens, without exception, can and ought to contribute to that common good in which individuals share so profitably to themselves."[33] Thus, rights are viewed in the context of the social nature of human beings. The encyclical does not merely address negative rights, such as the Lockean notion of a right to protect one's property. Rather, justice requires positive acts by various sectors of society that, rather than helping individual people, actively promote the common good.

The Contribution of *Quadragesimo anno*

Quadragesimo anno (*The Reconstruction of the Social Order*) was issued in 1931 by Pope Pius XI (papacy 1922–39) to honor the forty-year anniversary of *Rerum novarum.* Those decades had been filled with political and social tensions. By the thirties a worldwide economic depression had cast a cloud over the lives of untold millions. In Europe the left and right wings of political parties were gaining membership and power. It was also a time of religious intolerance in the Soviet Union and anticlerical movements in Mexico and Spain. Relations between the Vatican and the Italian Fascist regime were tenuous.

In *Quadragesimo anno*, Pius XI continues the discussion of justice, emphasizing the suffering that many people experience due to economic and social inequities. He argues that certain economic structures not only deny people basic necessities but treat people as means to an end, debasing the very dignity of personhood.[34] Not only is the distribution of public goods within society important, but so is the relationship between the person and society. This relationship is known as social justice.

Because social justice is concerned with the relationship of the individual and the common good, it guides societal institutions founded on the notion that human dignity itself is a social, rather than a private, concept.[35] Social justice governs the creation of public goods as well as the development of institutional organizations ordered to uphold the common good. It requires that individuals contribute to the creation and maintenance of these institutions while at the same time exercising their rights within their parameters. It also requires that governments guarantee and protect the rights of their citizens.

Pius XI makes another major contribution to Catholic social thought on justice with his discussion of the principle of subsidiarity. Although the principle was not cited in *Rerum novarum*, it has been part of almost every major Catholic social document since *Quadragesimo anno*. The principle of subsidiarity, rooted in the idea that the state exists for the well-being of the person and the family, holds that a higher or larger organization should not interfere in the lives of the individual or family if a lower or smaller organization can fulfill basic needs. In other words, intermediaries should provide assistance, if at all possible. Pius XI states it as follows:

> It is indeed true, as history clearly shows, that owing to the change in social conditions, much that was formerly done by small bodies can nowadays be accomplished only by large organizations. Nevertheless, it is a fundamental principle of social philosophy, fixed and unchangeable, that one should not withdraw from individuals and commit to the community what they can accomplish by their own enterprise and industry. So, too, it is an injustice and at the same time a grave evil and a disturbance of right

order to transfer to the larger and subordinate bodies. Inasmuch as every social activity should, by its very nature, prove a help to members of the body social, it should never destroy or absorb them.[36]

So, government has the power to intervene, but only as necessary to provide distributive and social justice. The theory of subsidiarity comes from the traditional Catholic thinking on "perfect" and "imperfect" forms of communities. The family and other voluntary types of associations are seen as neither self-contained nor complete in themselves. Thus, they are deemed imperfect societies. Recalling Thomas Aquinas, humans are thought to achieve their full humanity through a political society or state. The state, seen as having as its primary function to be the organizer of social life in its totality, is a perfect society—not perfect in the sense that any state is without flaws, but in the sense that only a state has the ability not only to promote but to protect the common good.[37]

Pius XI positions the principle of subsidiarity as the foundation upon which the social order should be reestablished, to halt socialism's excessive involvement of government in the lives of its citizens. He argues that action by a national government is warranted only when it can truly provide help to the smaller groups of individuals, families, and churches that make up society,[38] and only when "circumstances suggest or necessity demands."[39]

Building upon Augustine, Aquinas, and Leo XIII, Pius XI places a particularly strong emphasis on the relational aspects of justice. Human dignity exists within interdependent relationships. Justice is not merely distributive or commutative. Rather, it requires a system of social organizations that allow the person to develop fully, and this development can occur only within a mutually interdependent community. His endorsement of the principle of subsidiarity sets the stage for many subsequent debates the Catholic Church will have in attempting to define precisely the role of government in the lives of everyday citizens.

Pius XII and Human Dignity

Pope Pius XII, whose papacy spanned 1939–58, turned out to be very controversial. It was only two weeks after his coronation that Hitler invaded Czechoslovakia. In 1941 Italy declared war against Russia and the United States, putting the Vatican in an unenviable position. Pius XII tried to remain neutral between the opposing blocs, but today many questions still surround his actions during the war. The dominant question is this: Did Pius XII try enough (or at all) to stop Nazi atrocities against the Jews, the Serbs, the Poles, and other groups?[40] Regardless, during his pontificate Pius XII spoke more often and in a more systematic manner on "the moral roots of social, political, and economic order than had any of his predecessors."[41]

Pius XII thought that modern technology threatened human dignity. He argued that technology often subordinated the individual until he or she became "mere cogs in the various social organizations."[42] To counteract such consequences of modern technology, Pius proposed a vision of society as "a community of morally responsible citizens."[43] Moral theologian Charles Curran points out that this approach is a major change from that of Leo XIII, who saw no distinction between society and the state. Pius XII, though, saw the state as only one of several parts of society, the one that has the functions of defending rights and promoting freedom. Curran writes, "No longer is the state understood in terms of the relationship between *principes* and the untutored multitudes. The rulers are representatives of the people, and the people are responsible citizens."[44]

This represents a major development in justice theory. Now human dignity is intrinsically at the heart of the organization itself. It is no longer seen as a mere ideal for which governments should strive, but, as moral theologian David Hollenbach says, it becomes "a realizable moral imperative."[45] Human dignity is promoted through the satisfaction of certain conditions or human rights. In his Christmas Address of 1942, Pius XII suggests that human dignity consists of the following:

> respect for and the practical realization of the following fundamental personal rights: the right to maintain and develop one's corporal, intellectual and moral life and especially the right to religious formation and education; the right to worship God in private and public and to carry on religious works of charity; the right to marry and achieve the aim of married life; the right to conjugal and domestic society; the right to work, as the indispensable means toward the maintenance of family life; the right to free choice of a state of life, and hence, too, of the priesthood or religious life; the right to the use of material goods, in keeping with his duties and social limitations.[46]

Pius XII contends that every individual has the right to a governmental system that protects these rights. The role of government is to promote the common good through the defense of human rights. The common good thus consists of certain human rights founded on human dignity: "To safeguard the inviolable sphere of the rights of the human person and to facilitate the fulfillment of his duties should be the essential office of public authority. Does this not follow from the genuine concept of the common good which the State is called upon to promote?"[47] According to Hollenbach, Pius XII's vision of the common good and the role of government in promoting it reflects a vital distinction within the entire justice tradition. From Pius XII onward, human rights are inevitably linked to social interdependence,[48] the common good being defined by human rights, and human rights being socially interconnected.

Encyclicals of John XXIII

When Pius XII died in 1958, the seventy-six-year-old patriarch of Venice, Angelo Roncalli, was chosen as the next pope. To the surprise of many, he took the name John, which had not been used since the antipope John XXIII had been deposed at the Council of Constance in 1414 (because the antipope didn't "count," the modern John XXIII was carrying on the name from John XXII, whose papacy ended in 1334). This unusual choice of a name was the first sign of things to come. It is doubtful that many people foresaw the revolutionary changes that this vivacious Italian and his 1958–63 papacy would come to represent.

John XXIII's first encyclical on Catholic social teaching was *Mater et magistra (Christianity and Social Progress)*, issued in 1961 in commemoration of the seventieth anniversary of *Rerum novarum*. At the time of its writing, the world was a very different place from what it was during Leo XIII's pontificate. Technologies were rapidly changing; the automobile, the airplane, and television had radically altered communication and transportation. Typical education levels were rising, and political participation was increasing. Nations that had been colonized were seeking independence, based on claims of self-determinism. The stockpiling of atomic weapons and tensions between the Western world and communist Soviet Union and China created the Cold War. An overall realization of the complex interdependency of the modern world caused a new social awareness.

In *Mater et magistra*, John XXIII further defines the dignity of the person and its relationship to the common good. Essential to John XXIII's concept of human dignity is its emphasis on the existence of dignity within the actuality of social interdependence. This emphasis on what he calls "socialization" is much stronger than in prior encyclicals. John XXIII describes socialization as "the multiplicity of social relationships, that is, a daily more complex interdependence of citizens, introducing into their lives and activities many and various forms of association."[49] He goes on to note that this interdependence results in an increased involvement by public authorities in the personal lives of people in areas such as health care, education, career choice, and assistance for the disabled.

Within this context John XXIII asserts that human dignity and rights are the ultimate concern of the modern Catholic social tradition because "the cardinal point of this teaching is that individual men are necessarily the foundation, cause, and end of all social institutions."[50] The person, as mentioned earlier, is not the subject of economic and social life but, rather, is the *purpose* of it. This concept results in a stronger connection between human dignity and promoting the common good. John XXIII defines the latter as "the sum total of those conditions of social living, whereby men are enabled more fully and more readily to achieve their own perfection,"[51] equating the preservation and protection of human dignity with the attainment of social and economic rights.

On Holy Thursday 1963, only two months before his death, John XXIII issued *Pacem in terris (Peace on Earth)*. By then the world situation had become precarious. On the positive side, the United Nations had been founded in 1945, and in 1948 had issued its Declaration of Human Rights, affirming the dignity and worth of all people. This document had an important influence on John XXIII. Within the Catholic Church, it was a time of awakening. The Second Vatican Council opened on October 11, 1962, leading the Church on a journey during which it would examine its relationship with the modern world.

On the negative side, the Berlin Wall, a symbol of the ongoing Cold War, was erected in 1961. In October 1962, six months before John XXIII issued *Pacem in terris*, the Cuban Missile Crisis led to a tense standoff that many describe as the closest the world has ever come to a nuclear war. During the crisis John XXIII made a broadcast from the Vatican pleading for peace. Later Nikita Khrushchev, the Soviet premier, told the editor of the *Saturday Review* that "what the Pope has done for peace will go down in history."[52] In turn, Pietro Pavan, one of the drafters of *Pacem in terris*, acknowledged that the missile crisis inspired John XXIII to write the encyclical.[53]

Encyclicals are usually addressed to the world's Catholic bishops. *Pacem in terris*, however, was the first encyclical to be written to "all men of good will."[54] Its list of human rights is considered to be "the most complete and systematic list of these human rights in the modern Catholic tradition."[55] These rights derive from the dignity of the human person. They include rights related to sustaining life, such as the rights to food, clothing, shelter, health care, and assistance in cases of illness, old age, and unemployment; religious rights; rights regarding family life, including the rights to have a family and the necessities, such as economic and social opportunities, that are required for raising a family; economic rights, such as the rights to work, to a just wage, and to humane working conditions; and political rights, such as the rights to vote and to have access to a judiciary that one's rights be protected.[56] These rights come with corresponding duties. For example, the right to life has a duty to preserve it. The right to a decent standard of living is correlated with a duty to live it "becomingly."[57] Charles Curran argues that by including the corresponding duties, John XXIII avoids the pitfalls of individualism.[58]

The rights to which John XXIII refers were not new in Catholic thought. Yet the express manner in which he addresses each one is a departure from tradition. More importantly, *Pacem in terris* clearly defines human dignity in terms of human rights. Essential to the encyclical is the assertion that human dignity is totally interrelated with the political, social, and economic structures of society. It is not sufficient that institutions merely fulfill the basic requirements of human dignity. Rather, they *must* set up social, political, and economic structures that are actually ordered toward the promotion and protection of human dignity. By expressly stating a litany of rights, John XXIII also explicitly defines the universal common good in terms of rights language. He puts it as follows: "Like the common good of individual States, so too the universal common good cannot be determined except by having regard for the human person. Therefore, the public and universal authority, too, must have as its fundamental objective the recognition, respect, safeguarding and promotion of the rights of the human person."[59] With John XXIII human dignity, as well as the common good, comes to be defined by human rights. No longer is the person seen as a *part* of economic and social life. Instead, people are seen as the *purpose* of economic and social life. To promote human dignity, basic human rights must be met.

The Second Vatican Council and *Gaudium et spes*

On January 25, 1959, John XXIII announced that he was planning call an ecumenical council. At Vatican I, which had taken place almost one hundred years before, the major issue was the authority of the pope. John XXIII announced that the purpose of Vatican II was to promote the unity of all Christian people. The council, opened on October 11, 1962, became one of the most important events in the modern history of the Catholic Church. In all, it brought approximately twenty-five hundred of the world's top religious thinkers together for four three-month sessions over the course of four years. Sixteen documents were produced, covering a myriad of issues.

Vatican II made several major contributions to Catholic justice theory. One of the most important developments is reflected in the Church's change in methodology. Up until Vatican II, natural law was used as the major source for Catholic social principles. A natural law approach emphasized a classical worldview that stressed the universal and immutable. Natural law principles were used in a rather inflexible manner to address new situations and did not appreciate the fact that human existence is not static, that it is marked by social change and development.

The shift in methodology is reflected in *Gaudium et spes*, also known as the *Pastoral Constitution on the Church in the Modern World*. Written in 1965, it is one of the best-known and most controversial Vatican II documents. During Vatican II seventy draft documents were prepared by various appointed commissions. Most of these documents addressed internal issues within the Church. However, there was a movement, from within the ranks of bishops, calling for the Council to address not merely internal ecclesial issues but also issues external to the Church. *Gaudium et spes* is the first document from any council that was addressed to the people of the world: "Hence this Vatican Council . . . now addresses itself without hesitation, not only to the sons of the Church . . . but to the whole of humanity."[60] Its purpose is to bring the Church into dialogue with the rest of the world.

According to the document itself, its method is an examination of social and political issues "in light of the gospel and of human experience."[61] This signals a major movement away from a natural law methodology and toward an approach based on biblical revelation and historical consciousness. In fact, natural law is mentioned in only three places in the entire document. Instead, *Gaudium et spes* argues that social teaching cannot be understood without a consideration of biblical revelation. It uses Christology, biblical symbols, and biblical concepts such as creation, sin, and redemption to ground the Church's social mission.

Using this new methodology, *Gaudium et spes* gives us its second major contribution to Catholic social thought: a more nuanced understanding of human dignity. The document argues that human nature is conditioned by history. Humankind is developing, and this development is influenced by historical and social structures. Karl Rahner, a theologian who had great influence on *Gaudium et spes*, once wrote that our knowledge of human dignity "is itself a historically becoming process." As a result of this, "There is no zone of the person which is absolutely inaccessible to such influences from without."[62] By using a historical approach, the council attempts to understand humans within the context of salvation history.

Nevertheless, *Gaudium et spes* acknowledges that historicity is problematic because it creates a moral uncertainty: "Though mankind today is struck with wonder at its own discoveries and its power, it often raises anxious questions about the current trend of the world, about the place and role of man in the universe, about the meaning of his individual and collective strivings, and about the ultimate destiny of reality and of humanity."[63] On the one hand, people strive to be committed to religious values. On the other hand, constant historical and social changes create confusion about and anxiety over the definitions and limitations of such values. As a result, people are tempted either to shut themselves off from the world or to become slaves to historical relativism. Both of these responses are inappropriate and are, in essence, forms of human sinfulness because "man is split within himself."[64]

There is an appropriate response to the reality of historicity, however: the recognition that it is this very tension that makes us human. This human vulnerability to historical and social structures differentiates people from mere things.[65] A person's physical body and its relationship to the surrounding environment, the human relationships that develop, and the social structures needed to maintain such relationships are all imperative for personhood to exist.

Though, in essence, human dignity is recognized through historical and social structures, these structures must be ordered properly to ensure that it flourishes. As with earlier documents, the interdependence of people takes on a major role in *Gaudium et spes*, which gives interdependence even greater importance by arguing that it is an actual *characteristic* of human nature. Due to ever-increasing interdependence, social structures must be ordered to the common good, which is here defined as "the sum of those conditions of social life which allow social groups and their individual members relatively and ready access to their own fulfillment . . . and consequently involves rights and duties with respect to the whole human race."[66] These rights include rights to food, clothing, shelter, education, a family, employment, privacy, and religious freedom.[67] Furthermore, human dignity and the social nature of people require fundamental equality for all people, and "every type of discrimination, whether social or cultural, whether based on sex, race, color, social condition, language, or religion, is to be overcome and eradicated as contrary to God's intent."[68]

Finally, *Gaudium et spes* explicitly addresses the notion of stewardship, an implicit theme in many Catholic documents. The concept originates in Genesis 1:26, wherein humankind is called upon to have responsibility over God's creation: "Let them have dominion over the fish of the sea, and over the birds of the air, and over the cattle, and over every creeping thing that creeps upon the earth." In *Gaudium et spes*, the Council expressly acknowledges the importance of stewardship and attempts to define it. While discussing human dominance over nature, *Gaudium et spes* recognizes the interconnectedness of the modern world and asks the question "How should all these things be used?"[69] The document goes on to answer this question: "Man is able to love the things themselves created by God, and ought to do so. . . . Grateful to his Benefactor for these creatures, using and enjoying them in detachment and liberty of spirit, man is led forward into a true possession of the world, as having nothing, yet possessing all things."[70] Humankind has been entrusted to use God's creation in a prudent and unselfish manner. The world's resources are for the benefit of all, and thus a responsible use of these resources is a requirement of justice.

The Catholic Social Teaching of Paul VI

With the death of John XXIII, Pope Paul VI became the next pope (papacy 1963–78). He continued the work of Vatican II by overseeing the Council through its final sessions. During his pontificate Paul VI emphasized the importance of the Catholic Church in third world countries, where a large percentage of the population was Catholic. He appointed several cardinals from these countries and promoted regional synods of bishops to address issues that were important to people living in the third world. One such synod took place in Medellín, Colombia, in 1968, producing a significant theological statement on liberation theology. Also noteworthy was Paul VI's desire to travel to foreign countries. He was the first pope to travel throughout the world.

In March 1967 Paul VI issued his encyclical *Populorum progressio* (*The Development of Peoples*), which concentrated on development. Paul VI argues that the concept of development encompasses more than mere economic success. Rather, development is an integral notion that includes a full range of human capacities, including "freedom from misery; the greater assurance of finding subsistence, health, and fixed employment."[71] Paul VI suggests that there is a "Christian vision of development," wherein every human is created by God and therefore has a particular vocation and a right to fulfill his or her vocation. To be able to do so, certain human conditions must be met that contribute to human dignity, such as basic material necessities, access to education and culture, and freedom from oppressive social structures. Moreover, people have not only specific individual vocations but a social nature, which requires that their individual development be incorporated into the development of the community. In essence, every individual has the duty to contribute to the greater common good. Likewise, wealthier nations have the responsibility to help poorer nations achieve the integral development of their citizens. This responsibility is rooted in the concepts of human solidarity, social justice, and universal charity.[72]

What is most noteworthy in the encyclical in relation to the development of Catholic justice theory is Paul VI's understanding of how human dignity is further defined by integral development. Material well-being is integral to human dignity, not just useful to a person but necessary for complete human development. Material well-being is merely one facet of development, though. There are many social, intellectual, cultural, and religious conditions that must be met for a person to develop fully and achieve complete human dignity.

Paul VI's Apostolic Letter *Octogesima adveniens* (*A Call to Action*) was issued in 1971 in celebration of the eightieth anniversary of *Rerum novarum* and the tenth anniversary of *Mater et magistra*. Although it addresses new themes, such as urbanization and the environment, its main purpose is to clarify the relationship between the Church and governments.[73] *Octogesima adveniens* continues to refine the meaning of human dignity. Paul VI declares that equality and a right to participation are fundamental to human dignity: "While scientific and technological progress continues to overturn man's surroundings, his patterns of knowledge, work, consumption, and relationship, two aspirations persistently make themselves felt in these new contexts, and they grow stronger to the extent that he becomes better informed and better educated: the aspiration to equality and the aspiration to participation, two forms of man's dignity and freedom."[74]

Paul VI's claim that human dignity requires equality and a right to participation was a major progression in Catholic social thought. Prior to *Octogesima adveniens*, no Catholic document had established a right to participate in social, economic, and political decisions, and none had emphasized notions of equality so strongly. In fact, several earlier documents actually opposed equality.[75] Paul VI clearly rejects these prior teachings. He argues that all people have the right to be involved in the processes that influence their lives. One of the consequences of having these rights is that citizens will become more politically active. Paul VI states that the "Christian has the duty to take part . . . in the organization and life of political society."[76] Such a call for political action was quite radical in its day. Previous popes had actually discouraged political activism, even in view of the vast social, economic, and political injustices throughout history. For example, Leo XIII, who was more concerned with maintaining the political status quo, actually stated that the poor should be content with their lives, for their reward would be in heaven.[77] In *Octogesima adveniens*, Paul VI is more concerned with human rights than with maintaining political structures. He bases this argument on his notion that the lack of participation in society by large numbers of people is truly unjust. Christians actually have a duty to rectify this by creating the necessary venues enabling all to participate.[78]

The final major contribution to justice theory to come out of *Octogesima adveniens* is a teaching known as the preferential treatment of, or option for, the poor. It is a claim that the poor deserve special treatment. This idea was certainly not new to Catholicism, for it is rooted in scripture. In the Old Testament, the care of the weak and poor is a dominant theme. In the New Testament, in the Sermon on the Mount, Jesus announces that the poor are blessed. He identifies himself with the poor and oppressed. In his Second Letter to the Corinthians, Paul says that helping the poor of Jerusalem is an indication of love (8:8). In the Book of James, the poor are the chosen ones (2:5–6). Throughout modern church history, documents express compassion toward the poor and call for remedies.[79] Preferential treatment of the poor is a major element in liberation theology.

Yet, Paul VI was the first pope to emphasize the notion in a papal document. In *Octogesima adveniens* the plight of the poor takes on new meaning. Paul VI argues that the more fortunate are *required* to help the less fortunate and that this may necessitate that the more fortunate surrender some of their rights so the poor can live with dignity: "In teaching us charity, the Gospel instructs us in the preferential respect due to the poor and the special situation they have in society: the more fortunate should renounce some of their rights so as to place their goods more generously at the service of others."[80]

At the request of Paul VI, the world synod of bishops wrote its first social teaching document, *Justice in the World*, published on November 30, 1971. In its introduction, the synod writes, "Action on behalf of justice and participation in the transformation of the world fully appear to us as a constitutive dimension of the preaching of the Gospel."[81] The synod picks up on Paul VI's theme of development in *Populorum progressio* and makes a vital distinction. It argues that no single list of rights makes up the criteria for dignity. Instead, new ways of respecting dignity can emerge through analyses of economic, political, and social patterns of human interactions because there is a relational aspect to human dignity. The specifics of dignity can be ascertained only by viewing the individual person within his or her particular societal context and in relation to other people.[82] Moreover, the right to development is not merely an additional human right. On the contrary, the right to development is the primary requirement of human dignity. To achieve this right, people must be able to participate in economic, political, and social aspects of life. David Hollenbach suggests that the right to development "implies that all other rights are expressions of the claims of the person to be a self-determining agent, that is, they are expressions of claims to be a participant in the social, economic and political process."[83] The synod argues strongly that unjust social structures must be abolished because justice demands

> that the general condition of being marginal in society be overcome, so that an end will be put to the systematic barriers and vicious circles which oppose the collective advance toward enjoyment of adequate remuneration of the factors of production, and which strengthen the situation of discrimination with regard to access to opportunities and collective services from which a great part of the people are now excluded.[84]

That is, any social structure that impedes the ability to develop is a barrier to justice.

The U.S. Catholic Bishops and *Economic Justice for All*

The U.S. Catholic bishops' pastoral letter on Catholic social teachings and the U.S. economy, *Economic Justice for All*, took several years to complete. It was issued in 1986 after long and intense discussions took place within both the Catholic and the non-Catholic communities. Although written as a statement on economic matters, the pastoral letter makes a major contribution to the Catholic understanding of justice in its attempt to apply Catholic social teaching to substantive problems within the United States.

Building upon prior documents, the bishops ground their moral vision in the dignity of the human person in relation to others: "The dignity of the human person, realized in community with others, is the criterion against which all aspects of economic life must be measured."[85] One of the most important contributions the pastoral letter makes is defining a new measure of justice: justice by participation. Although the right to participation was a major theme of *Octogesima adveniens* and *Justice in the World*, it was not until *Economic Justice for All* that participation was actually deemed an *element* of social justice. The bishops state it as follows: "Basic justice demands the establishment of minimum levels of participation in the life of the human community for all persons. The ultimate injustice is for a person or group to be treated actively or abandoned passively as if they were nonmembers of the human race."[86] The pastoral letter describes this type of injustice as marginalization, defined as "exclusion from social life." Examples of such exclusion include political forms, such as the repression of people by the state, as well as an economic form, under the guise of poverty, wherein people are often excluded from sharing in resources. The bishops refer to these exclusions as "social sin" because social and economic inequities are created by humans who have free will and thus have the ability, and actually the responsibility, to correct them.[87]

In response to these exclusions, the pastoral letter contends that justice demands that "social institutions be ordered in a way that guarantees all persons the ability to participate actively in the economic, political, and cultural life of society."[88] This basic level of justice is defined by certain human rights to which all people are entitled. This is an important development in the Church's understanding of justice. The bishops make it clear that it is the responsibility of the community to ensure that all people are able to participate in societal structures: "Stated positively, justice demands that social institutions be ordered in a way that guarantees all persons the ability to participate actively in the economic, political, and cultural life of society."[89]

The document acknowledges that the degree of participation may legitimately vary between people but stresses that a "basic level of access" must be made available for everyone, as defined by certain human rights to which all people are entitled. Here the pastoral letter refers to John XXIII's list of human rights outlined in *Pacem in terris*. The bishops argue that these rights are necessary to protect human dignity. They ground this claim in the biblical tradition, which strongly "affirms the sacredness of every person as a creature formed in the image and likeness of God."[90] Moreover, covenant and community are essential in the Bible. Hence, human dignity can be realized and protected only through solidarity with others. The bishops, quoting *Gaudium et spes* in defining solidarity as the common good, describe the latter as "the sum of those conditions of social life which allow social groups and their individual members relatively thorough and ready access to their own fulfillment."[91]

After establishing the right of participation and grounding it in human dignity and the common good, the bishops emphasize the preferential treatment of the poor: "Everyone has special duties toward the poor and marginalized."[92] The bishops argue that such a commitment is deeply rooted in the biblical tradition. They suggest that in scripture the justice of a society is measured by the way in which its poor are treated. Throughout both the Old and the New Testaments, the needs of the poor and outcast are paramount, and "we are told that we will be judged according to how we respond to the hungry, the thirsty, the naked, the stranger."[93] Moreover, all are commanded to love one another as oneself. Therefore, the bishops conclude that the individual, the community, and the church are obligated to ensure that the poor are active participants in society.

John Paul II: Culture and Mercy

John Paul II was the first non-Italian elected pope in centuries. His 1978–2005 reign was marked by controversy. The most widely traveled of all popes, John Paul II brought his Christian message to millions throughout the world. He was extremely prolific as a teacher on justice, contributing three encyclicals that are imperative to the development of Catholic social teaching: *Laborem exercens* (*On Human Work*), *Sollicitudo rei socialis* (*The Social Concern of the Church*), and *Centesimus annus* (*On the Hundredth Anniversary of* Rerum novarum). Because these three documents contain essential teachings on market systems and the role of government, they will be covered in depth in the next chapter.

John Paul II's theology is of special relevance to this chapter. His anthropology influenced much of his subsequent social thought and is foundational to his development of an understanding of justice. His first encyclical, *Redemptor hominis* (*The Redeemer of Humankind*), issued in 1979, centers on redemption in Christ. God's love is made incarnate in Christ, and through his love, creation continues, and justice is revealed to us. Christ, therefore, is the measure of all humans. He is the model for all people. He is also the model for the Church, which must be an agent for redemption. To be so, the Church must respect the dignity of all people, for the human being is the "primary route that the Church must travel in fulfilling her mission: he is the primary and fundamental way for the Church."[94]

To promote human dignity, the Church must be located in the real world, in our culture, and working for humankind in a concrete way. This acknowledgment of culture is a major theme of John Paul II. Culture is a way of entering into human history where "the point of reference is transcendent, but the human lives in history, a history men and women are making, and the church is a historical actor, engaged and responsible."[95] John Paul II thus established a theological theme that both places the Church as an actor in the world and establishes Christ as the standard by which the Church analyzes and responds to the problems of the world.

In 1980 John Paul II issued the encyclical *Dives in misericordia* (*On the Mercy of God*), in which he links justice with mercy. He notes that through Christ, God is shown to us to be a God of mercy. He argues that the concept of mercy is not widely accepted in our modern time. In our age of science and technology, humans view themselves as "masters of the earth." Such a viewpoint leaves little room for mercy. Yet, precisely in these times people need the mercy of God.[96]

John Paul II uses the Parable of the Prodigal Son (Luke 15:11–32) to illuminate the Christian concept of mercy. He suggests that the mercy the father shows his son is an example of the biblical form of love known as agape. This kind of love restores dignity. It is never degrading to the one receiving it. John Paul II contends that many people see mercy as an unequal relationship between the one who gives mercy and the one who receives it. He suggests that this is wrong. In actuality, mercy establishes a relationship by which one party is happy to be the recipient of the dignity that mercy conveys because it brings him or her closer to God. The party offering the mercy is happy to help restore the other party's dignity. Therefore, an appreciation of human dignity stops the act of mercy from degrading the recipient: "The relationship of mercy is based on the common experience of that good which is man, on the common experience of the dignity that is proper to him."[97]

John Paul II goes on to link mercy with justice. Whereas justice emphasizes "objective and extrinsic goods," mercy brings dignity into relationships. Mercy therefore gives justice new content, which is expressed in forgiveness. Forgiveness is an avenue to reconciliation. Reconciliation is unifying and leads to solidarity. Hence, without mercy, justice is incomplete.[98] It is only through love and the act of reconciliation that human dignity can truly be restored.

Conclusion: What Is Justice?

Catholic social teaching on justice has evolved tremendously since the writings of Augustine and Aquinas. The development of Catholic social teaching shows that six central themes characterize the Catholic justice tradition.

1. *Human Dignity*. The starting place for assessing justice is human dignity. Because all people are created in the image of God, they have an innate and inalienable value or dignity. This dignity must be protected by recognizing the moral worth of the person. Everything is measured against the impact it will have on human dignity. The purpose of all institutions is to serve the people in ways that promote human dignity.

Human dignity is sometimes difficult to nuance because it is so dynamic. No single list of rights names all the criteria for dignity. New ways of understanding dignity can emerge through analyses of economic, political, and social patterns of human interactions, which continually change because human nature is conditioned by history. The specifics of human dignity can be ascertained only by viewing the individual person within his or her particular societal context and in relation to other people.

Nonetheless, the following conclusions about human dignity can be made. First, human dignity requires the assurance that people can develop a full range of capacities. This right to full human development is primary to dignity. It requires that the basic conditions necessary to enable persons to act as moral agents will be secured. These conditions, or rights, include, but are not limited to, the rights mentioned in *Pacem in terris*, such as the rights to food, clothing, shelter, medical care, education, religious expression, and so forth. Second, to achieve these rights, people must be able to participate in the economic, political, and social processes that affect their lives. Justice will not tolerate marginalization. Finally, respecting human dignity also requires that all people be viewed and treated as fundamentally equal. Any form of institutional or other discrimination is unjust.

2. *Social Interdependence*. The second principle of justice in Catholic social thought is an awareness of the ever-increasing interdependence of people and their communities in the contemporary world. This principle requires that justice cannot be understood apart from the reality of a labyrinth of social relationality. No one in the world lives a completely independent life. People are created by a triune God and are social beings who flourish within communities made up of social structures that are necessary for human existence. Human

dignity is totally interrelated with these political, social, and economic structures. Not only is the distribution of public goods within society important, but so is the relationship between the person and society. Within this context three forms of justice come into play. Distributive justice oversees the allotment of societal goods, commutative justice regulates dealings between individuals, and social justice governs the relationships between the individual and society.

3. *The Common Good.* The third principle of justice, in Catholic social teaching, is the notion that the good of the community is more important than the good of the individual. Because of the emphasis given the role of social interdependence, Catholic social thought requires positive acts by various sectors of society that, rather than privileging any single individual, actively promote the common good. The definition of "common good" is very nebulous. The term has been debated for decades and will continue to be debated. For the purposes of this book, I follow the definition of *Gaudium et spes*, which states that the common good is "the sum of those conditions of social life which allow social groups and their individual members relatively thorough and ready access to their own fulfillment, . . . and consequently involves rights and duties with respect to the whole human race."[99] In other words, the common good consists of certain human rights and duties that promote and protect dignity.

4. *Special Obligation to the Poor and Vulnerable.* Mandates to help the poor and other vulnerable people are found throughout the Gospel. From the early beginnings of Christianity, the Church has been committed to helping the less fortunate. Much of the Church's social teaching is aimed at creating a more humane world with just social structures. To create such a world, the particular circumstances and needs of the poor and vulnerable require special attention.

Due to difficult economic conditions, discriminatory practices, and other forms of marginalization, the poor and vulnerable are unable to develop in the full human sense, as required by the principle of promoting human dignity. Not only are they often excluded from participating in the political, economic, and social processes that affect their lives, but their basic material needs, such as sustaining levels of food and adequate shelter, are often not met. Under such conditions people cannot develop to their full capacities. Hence, justice requires that the Church, individuals, and society as a whole make special efforts to ensure that the poor and vulnerable are able to attain full human dignity.

5. *Stewardship.* Although stewardship has been discussed only briefly in this chapter, it is an important theme that will be developed later. Implicit in most Church documents is the underlying concept that all life and all the

earth's resources are gifts from God intended to benefit all of humankind. Thus, humankind has an obligation to care for these gifts and see that they are distributed in a fair and responsible manner.

6. *A Christian Interpretive Framework of Meaning.* Catholic social thought provides unique ways of understanding the world and avenues of meaning. A Christian interpretive framework of meaning is continually developing, being reinterpreted, and applied to contemporary issues. The central tenets of Christianity are the life, teachings, Passion, death, and resurrection of Jesus Christ. As John Paul II says, Christ, therefore, is the model for and the measure of all people. Justice must be interpreted through a Christian framework of meaning. Through Christ, God is shown to us to be a God of mercy. Without mercy, justice is incomplete.

I will continue to explore the uniqueness of the Christian interpretive framework of meaning and how it influences Catholic social thought on the just distribution of health care. Next I will examine Catholic social thought on capitalism and health care. With its often skeptical view of capitalism and advocacy of universal health care, the Church begs the question of whether market mechanisms should be applied to fund health care. It is only through the examination of the Church's views on capitalism and health care within the context of social justice that we can begin to assess whether the health care market can be moral.

Notes

1. Plato, *Republic of Plato*, Bk. IV, n. 433a.
2. Aristotle, *Nicomachean Ethics*, bk. 5.
3. Locke, "Second Treatise on Civil Government," n. 124.
4. Marx, "Critique of the Gotha Program," 531.
5. Nozick, *Anarchy, State, and Utopia*, 150.
6. Rawls, *A Theory of Justice*, 302.
7. Augustine, *City of God*, 72.
8. Ibid., 74.
9. Ibid., 470.
10. Ibid., 469.
11. Hollenbach, "Common Good Revisited," 81.
12. Augustine, *City of God*, 478.
13. Thomas Aquinas, "Summa Theologiae," vol. 2, I–II, q. 61, a. 5.
14. Ibid., III, q. 41, a. 1.

15. Ibid., II–II, q. 58, a. 1.

16. Ibid., I–II, q. 60, a. 3.

17. Ibid., II–II, q. 61, a. 1.

18. Ibid., I–II, q. 91, a. 1.

19. Ibid., I–II, q. 96, a. 1.

20. Ibid., I–II, q. 91, a. 2.

21. For an excellent discussion of the political and religious developments during this time, see Vidler, *Church in an Age of Revolution*, 45–189.

22. Mich, *Catholic Social Teaching and Movements*, 7.

23. International Theological Commission, "Communion and Stewardship," 233, 235–48.

24. Bokenkotter, *Church and Revolution*, 12–13.

25. See, for example, the discussion of Pius IX's "Syllabus of Errors" in Chadwick, *History of the Popes*, 168–81.

26. Leo XIII, *Rerum novarum*, n. 6.

27. Ibid., n. 5.

28. Ibid., n. 9.

29. Ibid., n. 12.

30. Ibid., n. 28.

31. Hollenbach, *Claims in Conflict*, 47.

32. Leo XIII, *Rerum novarum*, n. 34.

33. Ibid., n. 27.

34. Hollenbach, *Claims in Conflict*, 51.

35. Ibid., 55.

36. Pius XI, *Quadragesimo anno*, n. 79.

37. Hollenbach, *Claims in Conflict*, 159.

38. Ibid., 157.

39. Pius XI, *Quadragesimo anno*, n. 80.

40. The literature on Pius XII and his handling of the Nazi atrocities is mixed. Some is highly critical of him; see, for example, Cornwell, *Hitler's Pope*; Morley, *Diplomacy and the Jews*. Other books argue that in private the pope did much to help; see, for example, Rhodes, *Vatican in the Age of the Dictators*.

41. Hollenbach, *Claims in Conflict*, 56.

42. Pius XII, "Christmas Address, 1951," 156.

43. Ibid., 163.

44. Curran, *Moral Theology*, 181.

45. Hollenbach, *Claims in Conflict*, 59.

46. Ibid., 60.

47. Pius XII, "Pentecost Address, 1941," 31.

48. Hollenbach, *Claims in Conflict*, 61.

49. John XXIII, *Mater et magistra*, n. 59.

50. Ibid., n. 219.

51. Ibid., n. 65.

52. Cahill, *Pope John XXIII*, 205.

53. Himes, *Pacem in terris*, 697.

54. John XXIII, *Pacem in terris*, 131.

55. Hollenbach, *Claims in Conflict*, 66.

56. John XXIII, *Pacem in terris*, nos. 11–27.

57. Ibid., n. 29.

58. Curran, *Moral Theology*, 181.

59. John XXIII, *Pacem in terris*, n. 139.

60. Second Vatican Council, *Gaudium et spes*, n. 2.

61. Ibid., n. 46.

62. Rahner, "Dignity and Freedom of Man," 237, 242.

63. Second Vatican Council, *Gaudium et spes*, n. 3.

64. Ibid., n. 13.

65. Hollenbach, *Claims in Conflict*, 72–73.

66. Second Vatican Council, *Gaudium et spes*, n. 26.

67. Ibid.

68. Ibid., n. 29.

69. Ibid., n. 33.

70. Ibid., n. 37.

71. Paul VI, *Popularum progressio*, n. 6.

72. Ibid., n. 44.

73. Hollenbach, *Claims in Conflict*, 83.

74. Paul VI, *Octogesima adveniens*, n. 22.

75. See, for example, Leo XIII, *Humanum genus*, written in 1884, which rejected claims that people are equal.

76. Paul VI, *Octogesima adveniens*, n. 24.

77. Leo XIII, *Quod apostolici muneris*, n. 9.

78. Paul VI, *Octogesima adveniens*, n. 12.

79. See, for example, Leo XIII, *Rerum novarum*, n. 2; Pius XI, *Quadragesimo anno*, nos. 59, 112; John XXIII, *Mater et magistra*, nos. 68, 154.

80. Paul VI, *Octogesima adveniens*, n. 23.

81. Synod of Bishops, 1971, "Justice in the World," 289.

82. Hollenbach, *Claims in Conflict*, 87.

83. Ibid., 88.

84. Synod of Bishops, 1971, "Justice in the World," 290.

85. United States Catholic Bishops, "Economic Justice for All," n. 28.

86. Ibid., n. 77.

87. Ibid.
88. Ibid., n. 78.
89. Ibid.
90. Ibid., n. 79.
91. Ibid.
92. Ibid., n. 85.
93. Ibid., n. 16.
94. John Paul II, *Redemptor hominus*, n. 14.
95. O'Brien and Shannon, "Social Teaching of John Paul II," 348.
96. John Paul II, *Rich in Mercy*, n. 2.
97. Ibid., n. 6.
98. Ibid., n. 14.
99. Second Vatican Council, *Gaudium et spes*, n. 26.

2 Catholic Social Thought on Capitalism and Health Care

Capitalism, in one form or another, has existed as long as commercial activity has existed. Its main characteristic is that competition in a free market shapes the production and distribution of goods and services. Prior to Karl Marx, the system was simply known as commercial society or civil society.[1] Its opponents created the term *capitalism* to give it a negative connotation.

With its emphasis on trade and moneymaking, capitalism has a history of facing moral hostility. For example, in ancient Greece whatever enhanced the flourishing of the city-state was considered a civic virtue. The pursuit of personal monetary gain was often viewed with misgivings, as reflected in Plato's *Republic*, where Socrates remarks that "the more men value money-making, the less they value virtue."[2] The early Church fathers saw wealth as unjust because the wealth of one individual was thought to come at the loss of another. St. Jerome argued that the biblical description of wealth as "unjust riches" was, indeed, accurate because wealth has "no other source than the injustice of men, and no one can possess [unjust riches] except by the loss and ruin of others."[3] Augustine of Hippo was more direct when addressing wealth: "If one does not lose, the other does not gain."[4]

Yet, by the late Middle Ages, Europe saw the emergence of a more diverse economy. Cities grew, new ones developed, and new financial mechanisms were created. The Scholastic thinkers, such as Thomas Aquinas, took on a more nuanced approach toward trade by arguing that there is a difference between legitimate profits made from trade and immoral gain from usurious activity.[5] Though Catholic thinkers now put a more positive spin on commercial trade, the Church did not give people a free moral rein when it came to commerce. There were still the requirements of distributive justice to be met. Furthermore, it was believed that one should lead a virtuous life, and this could not be achieved by the pursuit of monetary profit. Greed was viewed as an impediment to salvation. In his 1697 treatise on usury, *Traité de Négoce et de L'Usure*, French cleric Father Thomassin writes,

> Those who accumulate possessions without end and without measure, those who are constantly adding new fields and new houses to their heritage; those who hoard huge quantities of wheat in order to sell at what to them is the opportune moment; those who lend at interest to the poor and rich alike, think they are doing nothing against reason, against equity, and finally against divine law, because, as they imagine, they do no harm to anyone and indeed benefit those who would otherwise fall into great necessity. . . . [Yet] if no one acquired or possessed more than he needed for his maintenance and that of his family, there would be no destitute in the world at all. It is thus this urge to acquire more and more which brings so many poor people to penury. Can this immense greed for acquisition be innocent, or slightly criminal?[6]

Of particular disdain to the Church was the lending of money to earn interest, or usury. For centuries, theologians and canonists continually redefined what constitutes usury. For example, utilizing different theories of money, they distinguished between loans and "partnerships."[7] Still, usurious activities were absolutely prohibited in Catholic countries by both civil and canon law into the eighteenth century. Pope Benedict XIV reaffirmed the prohibition against usury in his encyclical *Vix pervenit* in 1745.[8] As late as 1891, usury was still being discussed in papal documents. In that year Leo XIII condemned "rapacious usury" and compared it with greed.[9] It was not until the middle of the nineteenth century that the Vatican assured its followers that lending money at legal rates of interest was not going to jeopardize their souls.[10]

The economy of Europe had become a large commercial market by the eighteenth century. Commerce between Europe and Asia, Africa, and the Americas grew at a rapid pace. Urban areas grew quickly, and new modes of transportation opened the door for increased travel and trade. The fact that certain countries were wealthier than others caught the attention of Scottish moral philosopher Adam Smith, who wrote what is considered by many to be "the most important book ever written about capitalism and its moral ramifications."[11] Published in 1776, *An Inquiry into the Nature and Causes of the Wealth of Nations* reflects upon the economic success of eighteenth-century England. Smith notes that the average English laborer is better off economically than the elite classes in areas outside Europe, such as Africa. Why is this the case? There are two reasons: the division of labor and human self-interest. The specialized division of labor is essential to increased productivity because workers are more efficient when they do not have to switch back and forth between different tasks. The division of labor is possible because workers can exchange their labor and the products of their labor for other products. Smith calls this exchange "the market."[12]

Human self-interest drives the market. Smith argues that "the propensity to truck, barter, and exchange one thing for another" is part of human nature "and common to all men."[13] People are dependent upon one another to provide the items necessary for survival. This cooperation and assistance, however, does not come from the mere generosity of people. No, Smith insists, it must arise from self-interest:

> It is not from the benevolence of the butcher, the brewer, or the baker, that we expect our dinner, but from their regard to their own interest. We address ourselves, not to their humanity but to their self-love, and never talk to them of our necessities but of their advantages. Nobody but a beggar chooses to depend chiefly upon the benevolence of its fellow citizens.[14]

Economic self-interest benefits the whole community. Smith concludes that if people maximize their self-interest, products will be made more efficiently and more cheaply because it is in the best interest of both the producer as well as the community to do so. One of the unintended consequences of a profit motive and the resulting price mechanism is that the self-interest of individuals benefits the entire community. It has positive outcomes. Smith calls the unintended outcome of individual self-interest "an invisible hand" that promotes the good of society.[15]

The work of Adam Smith provides the foundation upon which capitalist economic theory is built. Since *An Inquiry into the Nature and Causes of the Wealth of Nations* was published, there has been rich and intense debate about market economies, and many theories expanding on Smith's work have been devised. For the purposes of this book, three terms need clarification. First, *liberalism* means different things around the world. In the United States, liberalism supports government that is actively involved in, and often intervenes in, the economy. The New Deal legislation of Franklin Roosevelt is considered liberal economic policy. In the rest of the world, though, *liberalism* basically means the opposite. It is akin to what *conservative* means in the United States and represents a belief in a reduced role for government, the support of economic freedom, and an emphasis on individual liberty. This notion of *liberalism* has its philosophical roots in thinkers such as John Locke and Adam Smith. So, when this book uses the term *liberalism*, I intend it to mean the philosophical position that supports less government, which is also the meaning the Catholic Church gives it.

Second, I am borrowing Jerry Muller's definition of *capitalism*: "a system in which the production and distribution of goods is entrusted primarily to the market mechanism, based on private ownership of property, and on exchange between legally free individuals."[16] And third, the term *market* means "the systematic exchange of labor and the products of labor" within a capitalistic system.[17]

Today nearly all developed countries have economic systems based on market mechanisms. Still, there are no pure capitalist economies in the world. All developed countries have varying degrees of government regulation. The United States, with the strongest economic system in the world, has had a love-hate relationship with government regulation. The first economic regulatory agency in the United States, the Interstate Commerce Commission, wasn't created until 1887. An era of antitrust legislation and suits followed, in which business monopolies and cartels were broken up for being anticompetitive. Following the onset of the Great Depression, the New Deal legislation of the 1930s and 1940s brought about sweeping regulations. For the next several decades, the United States saw strong regulatory agencies, and the robust antitrust tradition continued.

However, by the 1970s the intellectual movement known as the Chicago School of economics had caught fire. Named as such because several of its founders served on the economics faculty of the University of Chicago, the Chicago School emphasized a free market system and had little tolerance for government intervention in economics. In the early 1970s, the United States was hostage to high inflation, wage and price controls, and a bad recession. Deregulation and competition were seen as viable solutions to these serious economic problems. Beginning with the deregulation of the airline industry in 1978, the next twelve years also saw public utilities and the telecommunications industry deregulated, while many state and city governments privatized various public services, such as public transportation and garbage collection.[18]

Market competition has been reembraced. But what does the Catholic Church say about capitalism?

Capitalism and the Catholic Church

The *Catechism of the Catholic Church* says,

> The Catholic Church has rejected the totalitarian and atheistic ideologies associated in modern times with "communism" or "socialism." She has likewise refused to accept, in the practice of "capitalism," individualism and the absolute primacy of the law of the marketplace over human labor. Regulating the economy solely by centralized planning perverts the basis of social bonds; regulating it solely by the law of the marketplace fails social justice, for "there are many human needs which cannot be satisfied by the market."[19]

How did the Church arrive at this conclusion? What is there about capitalism and its market mechanisms that "fails social justice"? Why does the Catholic Church involve itself in economic matters at all?

Overview of the Church and Economic Thought

To understand the Church's interest in economic issues, one must first look to its anthropology. Its vision of earthly existence stems from Thomas Aquinas. Using Aristotelean philosophy, Aquinas argues that the natural end for all people is human flourishing. But, because of grace, everyone moves toward a supernatural end—friendship with God. The goal for humankind is to become virtuous, for it is through the virtues that people find their supernatural end.

Aquinas thought that political life is necessary for people to achieve their full humanity because people are social beings by nature. Thus, Catholicism sees the state as a natural institution arising out of human nature itself. Because Aquinas thought that society was organic and static, he did not see access to social structures as a problem. However, over the last one hundred years or so, the Church has come to recognize that society no longer functions in the organic model of Aquinas's time. With the massive urbanization and industrialization of Western Europe and the United States, and with the more recent technological revolution, the Church has become critical of what it considers unjust social structures, economic systems among them.

Another reason the Church concerns itself with economic matters is that, whereas economics is often assessed by levels of efficiency and consumer choices, the Church assesses all social structures, including economic systems, from its own perspective, especially that characterized by the themes listed at the end of chapter 1, offering a unique point of view on economic issues that is not found within the field of economics itself. Thus, Catholic social teaching offers an important perspective not found in other disciplines.

Catholic theologian Thomas Massaro points out that the Church does not ally itself politically with any particular system. Its key loyalties are to theological concepts and values, rather than to partisan politics or economic ideologies.[20] Although Catholic social teaching is critical of aspects of all economic systems, for the purposes of this book I shall focus on its critique of capitalism. Before beginning that task, it is important to understand that the major tenet of the Church's teaching on economic systems is that they affect all in society. They are not, therefore, meant to help merely a few people or a majority of people. The U.S. bishops make this point brilliantly: "We judge any economic system by what it does *for* and *to* people and by how it permits all to *participate* in it. The economy should serve people, not the other way around."[21] An economic system must promote the common good of all people.

Papal Documents

The Church's critique of capitalism begins with Leo XIII's *Rerum novarum*. As discussed in chapter 1, Leo XIII acts as an advocate for workers. He affirms the Church's position that justice, not market mechanisms, should govern workers' wages and working conditions.[22] In *Quadragesimo anno*, Pius XI endorses Leo XIII's position that people have a right to own private property. Still, Pius XI argues that to overcome the extreme individualism, and contrary to the distaste for government regulation that capitalism proclaims, the state has the right to regulate the ownership of property to ensure that it is used to promote the common good.[23]

In *Mater et magistra*, John XXIII continues the economic tradition of Leo XIII and Pius XI. He argues that the distribution of goods and working conditions of employees, rather than the levels of productivity, are the most important factors in judging an economic system to be just.[24] In *Pacem in terris*, John XXIII uses the term "economic rights" to designate several rights specifically related to economic activities. Among economic rights, he mentions the right to work, the right to safe working conditions, and the right to a just wage.[25]

Paul VI presents a more severe critique of capitalism. In *Populorum progressio* he criticizes the key elements that are essential to capitalism:

> But it is unfortunate that on these new conditions of society a system has been constructed which considers profit as the key motive for economic progress, competition as the supreme law of economics, and private ownership of the means of production as an absolute right that has no limits and carries no corresponding social obligation. This unchecked liberalism leads to dictatorship rightly denounced by Pius XI as producing "the international imperialism of money." One cannot condemn such abuses too strongly by solemnly recalling once again that the economy is at the service of man. But if it is true that a type of capitalism has been the source of excessive suffering, injustices, and fratricidal conflicts whose effects still persist, it would also be wrong to attribute to industrialization itself evils that belong to the woeful system which accompanied it.[26]

Paul VI makes it clear that it is a *type* of capitalism that is unjust; he does not offer a blanket condemnation of capitalism. It is capitalism's primary values of economic efficiency and individualism to which he objects, because they represent an "erroneous affirmation of the autonomy of the individual in his activity, his motivation, and the exercise of his liberty."[27]

However, it is John Paul II who provides the most nuanced critique of capitalism. He addresses this issue in three encyclicals. In *Laborem exercens* (*On Human Work*, 1981), he uses his theory of labor as a basis for critical consideration of economics. Written to analyze the question of human work, John Paul II attests that human work "is a key, probably the essential key, to the whole social question."[28] He argues that all people are designed to work and, therefore, by taking part in work, they largely realize their human potential. There are two meanings associated with the term *work*. The objective meaning refers to the products made by labor, such as manufactured goods and technology. The subjective meaning refers to the realization of human fulfillment that results from work. The subjective meaning of work has priority over the objective meaning of work because work is necessary to reach full human potential. Hence, work is for the person, rather than the person is for work. This conclusion provides us with a key ethical criterion: Economic systems should be evaluated according to the impact they have on workers, instead of the impact they have on production or capital.

John Paul II critiques capitalism with this ethical criterion. The problem with capitalism is that it places a priority on the objective meaning of work over the subjective meaning of work. Under such a system people are regarded as commodities: "Man is treated as an instrument of production."[29] The priority of the objective meaning of work over the subjective meaning of work is "the error of early capitalism," which occurs whenever human labor is viewed only according to its economic purpose.[30] John Paul II calls this an "error of materialism," in that such an economic system gives priority to material or capital over the importance of the human or the personal. The error of materialism occurs because of greed, which places great importance on capital while basically ignoring the means by which this capital was produced, human labor.[31]

John Paul II uses the priority of labor over capital to nuance the Church's understanding of private property. While acknowledging the usefulness of private property, he also criticizes the notion within capitalistic systems that the ownership of private property is an absolute right. He suggests that "the position of 'rigid' capitalism continues to remain unacceptable, namely the position that defends the exclusive right to private ownership of the means of production as an 'untouchable dogma' of economic life."[32] Instead, he contends, the ownership of the means of production, whether private, public, or collective, must serve labor.[33]

John Paul II continues his critique of capitalism in *Sollicitudo rei socialis* (*The Social Concern of the Church*, 1987). Again he discusses private property, which must serve the common good. He acknowledges that private property is necessary but adds that "the goods of this world are *originally meant for all*," so private property is "under a 'social mortgage' which means that it has an intrinsically social function, based upon and justified precisely by the principle of the universal destination of goods."[34] John Paul II also notes the lack of development in many developing countries. He blames both the communist and the Western blocs for causing the poverty and underdevelopment in so many parts of the world. Regarding the West, John Paul II points a finger at the "principles of liberal capitalism," which, with its unique view of human nature, promotes an "*all-consuming desire for profit*," which is opposed to both "the will of God" and "the good of neighbor."[35] He concludes that such an economic system results in "real forms of idolatry: of money, ideology, class, technology."[36]

John Paul II's final social ethics encyclical, *Centesimus annus* (*On the Hundredth Anniversary of* Rerum novarum, 1991), provides the Church with not only a strong critique of capitalism but some important guidelines for judging market economies. The encyclical, written in light of the vast political and economic changes across Eastern Europe and other parts of the world in 1989, attempts to analyze these changes. In keeping with the social teaching tradition, John Paul does not endorse any particular economic system. Instead, he attempts to answer the following question: "Can it perhaps be said that, after the failure of communism, capitalism is the victorious social system, and that capitalism should be the goal of the countries now making efforts to rebuild their economy and society?"[37] John Paul II begins by reasserting his position in *Laborem exercens*: The error of capitalism is found in its incorrect prioritization of capital over labor, which turns the human worker into a mere commodity.[38]

He goes on to criticize capitalism on several grounds. First, it ignores the universal "destination of goods" principle.[39] Second, it does not provide properly for the treatment of workers.[40] Third, capitalism has a negative effect on the relationship between the state and its citizens. By limiting the role of the state in economic matters, the state in essence becomes an advocate for the rich while ignoring the needs of the poor.[41] Finally, John Paul II criticizes the "phenomenon of consumerism," which arises because of a mistaken emphasis on "having," rather than on "being." He argues that people should focus on spiritual goods and the common good of the community, instead of acquiring goods that satisfy "artificial needs."[42]

Still, John Paul II does find some positive attributes in capitalism. It is based on human freedom and knowledge and contains an implicit duty to use that freedom and knowledge responsibly.[43] He acknowledges that such a system is very efficient and responsive to many human needs. The ideal economic system for John Paul II would retain these characteristics, while at the same time—"within a strong juridical framework," an administrative structure combining elements of the state and the private sector—it would be supportive of the dignity and rights of workers and encourage social participation by all members of society.[44]

To establish such a system, John Paul II first looks to the state, which "has the task of determining the juridical framework within which economic affairs are to be conducted."[45] Then he suggests that both the state and the private sector should ensure adequate wage levels, humane working conditions, and provide for the proper training of workers.[46] John Paul II points out that there are "many human needs" that cannot be met by the market and "it is a strict duty of justice and truth not to allow fundamental human needs to remain unsatisfied, and not to allow those burdened by such needs to perish."[47] Thus, market economies have an important role, but they must be supplemented by government and the private sector to ensure that human dignity is protected and that all people have an opportunity to participate fully in society.

The Church and Economics in the United States

The United States is a unique case. It is perhaps the strongest example of capitalism in the world. With its reverence for independence, individualism, self-sufficiency, and material wealth, the United States incorporates the virtues of the market economy.

The relationship between the United States and the Catholic Church is also unique, particularly in comparison with Europe. In the United States, the Church has never been identified with political power, as it had been in Europe. Moreover, there is no state religion, and, to the contrary, there exists a strong legal tradition of separation of church and state. And although there are many Catholics in the United States, they began as immigrant minorities and were originally associated with the working classes. For these reasons, the Catholic Church in the United States has often identified with the economic problems of its members.

The U.S. bishops first published a major opinion on economics at the end of World War I, in 1919. The document, *Social Reconstruction: A General Review of the Problems and Survey of Remedies*, was drafted by Monsignor John Ryan, an influential professor of social ethics at Catholic University of America.[48] In this document the U.S. bishops called for a just wage, better working conditions, and the right to form unions.[49] In that same year, the National Catholic Welfare Council (its name changed to the National Catholic Welfare Conference [NCWC] in 1922) was established as a successor to the National Catholic War Council, which had served to oversee and unite American Catholics during WWI.[50] For the next four decades, the U.S. bishops expressed their voice through the NCWC. One of the original divisions of the NCWC was the Social Action Department. Originally chaired by Monsignor Ryan, who led the department until 1945, its first publication was the *Bishops' Program of Social Reconstruction*. The document supported a minimum wage, social security, welfare for the poor, and unions. During the Depression the NCWC's administrative committees severely criticized the market system as "callous and autocratic possessors of wealth and power who use their poison and the riches to oppress their fellows."[51]

Throughout the 1930s and 1940s, the NCWC took strong economic stances. It became a hotbed of social activism. During the New Deal years, Ryan spoke in support of unions, strong government programs for economic relief and reform, and the National Industry Recovery Act. The NCWC started Labor Schools and Schools of Social Action, which trained many lay activists.[52] It continued its social activism until 1966, when, as a part of a general restructuring, it changed its name to become the National Conference of Catholic Bishops (NCCB) and the U.S. Catholic Conference (USCC). The Social Action Department became the Department of Social Development. In 2001 the NCCB and the USCC were combined to form the U.S. Conference of Catholic Bishops.

With the publication of *Economic Justice for All* in 1986, the bishops issued a firm statement on economics. The pastoral letter does not expressly critique capitalism. Rather, it addresses specific problems with the economic system in the United States and makes recommendations on how to make the system more just. Yet, a critique of capitalism can be drawn out by scrutinizing the bishops' views on problems with the economic system and by analyzing their recommendations for solving these problems.

Economic Justice for All was written to "discover what our economic life must serve, what standards it must meet."[53] To determine these standards, the letter establishes certain moral principles that should govern economic life. These six moral principles can be summarized as follows: All economic decisions and institutions must protect human dignity; human dignity can be promoted only through the community; all people have a right to take part in the economic life; we have a special obligation to the poor and vulnerable; human rights, including economic rights, are the minimum standard for human existence; and society, acting through public and private sectors, has a responsibility to protect human rights.[54]

The pastoral letter emphasizes several "urgent" problems associated with the United States' economy, including a high unemployment rate, increasing rates of poverty, and a growing disparity in income. The bishops then ask the following questions: "Does our economic system place more emphasis on maximizing profits than on meeting human needs? Does our economy distribute its benefits equitably or does it concentrate power and resources in the hands of a few? Does it promote excessive materialism and individualism?"[55] The critique of capitalism is found in these questions. The bishops are suggesting that capitalism emphasizes making profits over meeting human needs, causes an unjust distribution of wealth, and promotes excessive materialism and individualism.

What are the bishops' recommendations for dealing with these consequences of capitalism? Noting that the Church's teaching "rejects the notion that a free market automatically produces justice,"[56] they offer the following four objectives: to make the needs of the poor the highest priority; to increase the active participation in economic life by the marginalized; to invest resources specifically to help the poor; and to evaluate economic and social policies in view of their impact on family life.[57] They suggest that certain specific actions can help achieve these objectives, such as supporting labor unions and using private property to promote the common good. They also encourage government to enact legislation to create a tax system that is more equitable, set up work programs for the poor, and establish more successful welfare programs.[58]

The Catholic Right and Left: Other Opinions on Capitalism

Since Vatican II there has been a wide range of Catholic opinions on capitalism. From neoconservativism to liberation theology, economics is a controversial subject.

One of the best-known neoconservative Catholic thinkers in the United States is Michael Novak, who has written several books endorsing the merits of capitalism. Novak argues that the United States is a wonderful example for the rest of the world because it combines a strong sense of individualism with a communitarian spirit. He is an advocate of what he calls "democratic capitalism," which consists of three separate systems: an economic system based on the market, a political system founded on individual rights, and a cultural and moral system inspired by freedom and justice. Each system should be independent of the others. Novak argues that the Church, in its critique of capitalism, unfairly imposes standards from the cultural and moral system onto the economic system.[59] He suggests that there is a strong link between democracy and a market economy, for a "political democracy is compatible in practice only with market economy."[60]

Novak defends capitalism against the criticisms of the Church. He argues that capitalism is the best system to help the poor and contends that inefficient distribution of wealth is not the cause of poverty. Rather, it is a failure to produce enough wealth.[61] One of the major reasons this failure exists is because of political systems that "penalize the economic behavior of economically creative citizens."[62] To illustrate his argument, he looks to Latin America, where "it's almost impossible for poor people to start businesses of their own, because the fees and the bribes that have to be paid are so high."[63] Because the democratic system, which goes hand in hand with capitalism, consists of a system of checks and balances, including a competitiveness that prevents a small group of individuals from abusing a disproportionate share of economic power, Novak suggests that many of the bad characteristics of human nature, such as greed, are neutralized.[64] Furthermore, he finds virtue in a key aspect of capitalism that most Church documents deem problematic: the notion that capitalism functions as a result of self-interest. Novak suggests that this is a positive feature of capitalism because it emphasizes "the humbleness of the human race" and therefore "accepts human beings in their sinfulness rather than in their grandeur."[65]

Representing the other end of the spectrum of Catholic thought on capitalism is liberation theology. There is no single liberation theology. The best-known liberation theology arose out of Latin America in the 1960s, during enormous political and economic changes. In 1959 Castro had taken over Cuba. President John F. Kennedy inaugurated his Alliance for Progress in 1961 to stimulate economic growth, stabilize price levels, increase literacy, and increase low-cost housing. The program was not particularly effective, and although some progress was made, overall it was considered a failure.[66] In 1964 a military coup in Brazil overthrew democratic government, a situation that would last twenty years. Many governments in Latin America began to employ security forces that used brutal tactics to maintain political control. University students became attracted to Marxism, and several Catholic theologians, such as Dom Hélder Camera of Brazil, Camilo Torres of Colombia, and Gustavo Gutiérrez of Peru, began to denounce poverty and capitalism and call for social change.[67]

There are several assumptions that are shared among liberation theologies. Advocacy and praxis (putting theory into action) are very important. Whereas many other types of theology are deductive, reasoning from the general to the specific, liberation theology uses the opposite approach, induction, in proposing a unique view of the relationship between theory and praxis: Theory is shaped by praxis as much as praxis shapes theory. According to Juan Luis Segundo, "a liberation theologian is one who starts from the opposite end. His suspicion is that anything and everything involving ideas, including theology, is ultimately bound up with the existing social situation in at least an unconscious way."[68] Liberation theology also uses social analysis to examine historical locations of a particular group of people and emphasizes human experience and justice.

Liberation theology's critiques of capitalism are abundant. Key to these critiques is liberation theology's use of the perspective of the poor and oppressed as a starting point. The early critiques of capitalism within a liberation theology context came out of a conference held by the bishops of Latin America in Medellín, Colombia, in 1968. The bishops wrote three documents, one each on peace, justice, and poverty. Together they make up what are known as the Medellín Documents. These texts took a firm stand declaring that the Church should focus on helping the poor organize to attain justice. They contended that Latin America suffers from "tensions between classes" and "a marked bi-classicism," which constitute sinful structures.[69] They argued that capitalism compromises human dignity because it "takes for granted the primacy of capital, its power and its discriminatory utilization in the function of profit-making." The bishops called for a major transformation to create "a just social system."[70]

The conference at Medellín fueled the liberation theology movement. Criticisms of capitalism by liberation theologians became widespread. José Míguez Bonino wrote,

> Capitalism creates in the dependent countries (perhaps not only in them) a form of human existence characterized by artificiality, selfishness, the inhuman and dehumanizing pursuit of success measured in terms of prestige and money, and the resignation of responsibility for the world and for one's neighbor. . . . This sham culture kills in the people even the awareness of their own condition of dependence and exploitation, it destroys the very core of their humanity.[71]

In *A Theology of Liberation*, Gustavo Gutiérrez quoted from Medellín Documents when he argued that "private ownership of capital leads to the dichotomy of capital and labor, to the superiority of the capitalist over the laborer, to the exploitation of man by man. . . . We must hence opt *for social ownership of the means of production.*"[72] There are many other criticisms of capitalism by liberation theologians, but one theme prevails: Capitalism, with its emphasis on the primacy of money and profit, contributes to poverty, the exploitation of people, and other injustices causing immense suffering.

The Vatican has been highly critical of liberation theology. In 1979 John Paul II visited the Latin American bishops' conference held at Puebla, Mexico. He affirmed the Church's mission to help the poor and marginalized and to work on behalf of justice. He reaffirmed the Church's position that the private ownership of property carries with it a social obligation. But he also criticized liberation theology for the politicization, particularly leftist political activism, of Catholic theology by arguing, "It is a mistake to state that political, economic, and social liberation coincide with the salvation in Jesus Christ."[73] After Puebla, John Paul II appointed several conservative bishops to replace those who supported liberation theology and disciplined liberation theologian Leonardo Boff for certain claims found in his book *Church: Charism and Power.*[74]

Summary: The Church's Critique of Capitalism

Many representatives of the Catholic Church are highly critical of capitalism, arguing that it is morally limited because it is does not meet the basic principles of justice. Using the six principles from chapter 1, these critiques of capitalism can be summarized as follows.

1. Capitalism threatens *human dignity* in two major ways. First, it often creates situations in which the person is commodified, used as a means to make money solely for the sake of profit, which results in the exploitation of the person. This pattern of exploitation was particularly notable during the industrial revolution of the eighteenth century, when working conditions were often inhumane, wages were barely enough for subsistence, and workers had virtually no right of recourse against their employers. Today this type of exploitation still exists.

One example of human commodification is child labor. In Latin America, for example, where half of the population lives in poverty, children are often expected to contribute to their families' meager incomes. Approximately 27.4 million Latin American children under the age of fourteen work.[75] Often these children are unable to attend school. Their jobs include street vending, housekeeping, and hauling produce to markets. There are many risks associated with child labor, including exposure to extreme temperatures, physical stress on developing bone structures, and sexual harassment.[76] Although there are many factors that contribute to child labor, it can be argued that the unequal distribution of income resulting from capitalistic monetary policies contributes to the creation of an economic system that commodifies children.

A second major threat to human dignity associated with capitalism is an extreme emphasis on profit. The profit motive is essential to capitalism, but it encourages such vices as greed and materialism. These vices, in turn, chip away at human dignity because when greed and materialism are motivating factors, people become a means to acquire material goods. Remember that Catholic social thought teaches that all people have a right to full human development and that this right can be achieved only if all people can meet the basic conditions that enable them to participate fully in social, economic, and political processes that affect their lives. Greed and materialism often result in conditions where people cannot meet basic material needs, such as adequate food, shelter, and clothing.

2. Another critique of capitalism is that it fails to recognize and encourage the *social interdependence* of people. With its excessive emphasis on individualism and self-interest, capitalism ignores the fact that human flourishing requires reciprocal cooperation between people. David Hollenbach argues that the disparity in incomes and lifestyles between classes in the United States results in a state of unequal interdependence between people "who hold very different amounts of power. . . . In a relation of unequal interdependence, one of the partners has the power to make things happen while the other partner lacks such power."[77] In their most extreme form, unequal relationships manifest themselves in the shape of slavery, but wherever there is disparity in income or social status, there is unequal interdependence. Capitalism promotes such disparities. Hollenbach argues that in a system of unequal interdependence, those who are subordinate "do not share actively in governing themselves but must simply cope with decisions made by another."[78]

Another way capitalism fails to recognize the social interdependence of people is that it often ignores the social purpose of private property. Although property can help its owner meet his or her material needs, Catholic social thought argues that it has a broader, multidimensional social function. John Paul II calls this concept a "social mortgage," meaning that private property should be used to serve and benefit everyone, not just the property owner.

3. Capitalism, with its stress on individualism, does not always promote the *common good*. Capitalism encourages people to act out of their personal self-interest rather than in the interest of others. Catholic social thought contends that the good of each person is connected to the good of other people. Each person has an obligation to contribute to the common good, so that all people, not merely certain individuals, can flourish.

Another critique Catholic social thought makes is that capitalism restricts the role of government. As noted earlier, Catholic social thought sees government as a positive institution that is necessary for intervening in social, political, and economic sectors to ensure that the common good is protected and promoted, not only the good of some individuals. For these reasons John Paul II insists that capitalism should operate only through a strong juridical framework.

4. Catholic social thought emphasizes that we all have a *special obligation to the poor and vulnerable*. Adam Smith's theory of capitalism suggests that one of the unintended consequences of the profit motive and the resulting price mechanism is that the self-interest of individuals would benefit the entire community. This "invisible hand" would promote the good of the whole society.

However, the invisible hand does not seem to be doing its job. In contemporary capitalist countries, huge disparities in wealth are found, resulting in severe poverty. For example, in the United States, a country that prides itself on its market economy, 12.7 percent of the entire population, 37 million people, lived at or below the poverty level in 2004.[79] In Latin America, where the invisible hand is often relied on to drive economies, the statistics are much more alarming. Approximately 44 percent of the area's population lives on less than $2.00 per day.[80] In Mexico the wealthiest 20 percent of the population receives 58 percent of the national income, and the poorest 40 percent receives only 11 percent.[81] The existence of so much poverty is evidence that market economies do not sufficiently protect the poor and vulnerable.

5. Capitalism challenges Catholic social thought on the importance of *stewardship*. The best example of this is the Church's notion of a social mortgage: Private property is necessary, but material goods are gifts from God meant for all to use. So, we have an obligation to ensure that people have access to goods and that these goods benefit all of humankind. Capitalism values private property, but because of its emphasis on individualism, capitalism views private property as benefiting solely the owner of the property and encourages the owner to do whatever he or she wishes with the property, without regard to others.

6. Finally, much of Catholic social teaching on capitalism arises out of a *Christian framework of meaning*. The belief that people are all created in the image of God is the foundation for the requirement of human dignity. The belief that God created the world and all of its resources for the benefit of all people requires that we should use goods accordingly. Christians are called to imitate the life and teachings of Jesus Christ. The parables and the Sermon on the Mount provide a biblical foundation for Catholic social thought's emphasis on showing mercy, charity, and compassion toward all people, especially the poor and vulnerable. Capitalism often falls short of these goals.

Catholic Social Thought and Health Care

The Roman Catholic Church has a long tradition of involvement in medical issues through two main avenues, moral theology and pastoral medicine. As early as the fifteenth and sixteenth centuries, the obligations of physicians appear in some of the confessors' manuals.[82] The manuals themselves were not devoted specifically to medical issues. Nonetheless, these topics arose under certain headings.[83] For example, regarding the fifth commandment ("Thou shalt not kill"), issues concerning abortion, euthanasia, and sterilization are discussed. There is a special section on the obligations of physicians and other medical personnel, which includes the duties to follow safe medical practices, avoid harmful practices, and obtain the proper skills necessary for the profession.[84]

Another source of the long relationship between medical ethics and Catholic theology is the tradition of pastoral medicine, which investigates the interface of medicine and theology.[85] In pre-Christian times healing was most often identified with the priest, the job of healing sick people being practiced by "holy men." Hippocrates was the first person to establish medicine as a skill based on rational observation, diagnosis, and prescription, thereby distinguishing healing from a priestly ministry.[86] As Christianity spread across the Roman Empire, the teachings of the Gospel influenced the physician to see himself and the profession as a vocation "to be a Christlike service of salvific healing."[87] Hence, medical treatment must be equitable, available for free to the poor, and include spiritual counseling.

Up until the first half of the seventh century, the majority of physicians were laymen. With the collapse of the Roman Empire, though, Christian structures began to take over medicine. In the sixth century, monasteries began to care for the ill, and between the seventh and twelfth centuries, lay doctors were rare.[88] However, this began to change in the twelfth and thirteenth centuries, with the establishment of a large medical school at Salerno, Italy, the inclusion of medical faculties at urban universities, and a series of ecclesiastical decrees that forbade the practice of medicine by religious orders.[89] Although ordained people continued working in the medical profession throughout the Middle Ages and into modern times, the profession became more and more dominated by laypeople.

In the United States, several Catholic theologians were essential to the development of medical ethics. The first American work on morals in medicine, *Moral Principles and Medical Practices: The Basis of Medical Jurisprudence*, was written in 1897 by Charles Coppens, SJ, a professor at Creighton Medical College. The book deals with medical jurisprudence, or the formal study of medicine. It treats subjects such as abortion and the duties of the physician in view of philosophical and theological principles. In the early 1920s Jesuit ethics professor Henry Spalding wrote a book on ethics for nurses and nursing students. He also added three chapters to Coppens's work, dealing with issues such as euthanasia and birth control. During the 1940s and 1950s the works of Augustinian priest Charles McFadden were widely read. His book *Medical Ethics*, first published in 1946, was a popular textbook for Catholic medical students, nurses, and seminarians; the five revised and updated editions have been published since then. His work has been highly influential in establishing medical ethics as an independent discipline.[90]

One of the most influential Catholic medical ethicists in the United States in the 1950s was Gerald Kelly, SJ. He wrote many articles for the journal *Hospital Progress* and greatly influenced the writing of the original *Ethical and Religious Directives for Catholic Hospitals* (the 4th edition, with the United States Bishops as author, is titled *Ethical and Religious Directives for Catholic Health Care Services*). Throughout the 1950s and into the 1960s, several textbooks and manuals addressing medical issues were written by Catholics.[91]

With the papacy of John XXIII and his *Pacem in terris* (1963), health care was deemed a right in Catholic social thought. This opened the door for further thinking on medical issues and health care. John XXIII viewed as human rights both medical care and security when facing sickness: "Beginning our discussion of the rights of man, we see that every man has the right to life, to bodily integrity, and to the means which are suitable for the proper development of life; these are primarily food, clothing, shelter, rest, medical care, and finally the necessary social services. Therefore a human being also has the right to security in cases of sickness."[92]

In the 1960s booming technological advances in medicine and questions surrounding research with human subjects created intense controversies concerning such issues as prolonging life, eugenics, and abortion. Conferences were held, and eventually bioethics institutes were established, to address these questions. These developments gave birth to the field of bioethics.

Catholic theologians—such as the late Richard McCormick, Charles Curran, Philip Keane, Margaret Farley, Lisa Cahill, and Edmund Pellegrino, the current chairman of the President's Council on Bioethics—have continued the Church's tradition of addressing questions of medical ethics.

The Catholic Health Association

The Catholic Health Association of the United States and Canada was established in 1915 "for the promotion and realization of progressively higher ideals in the religious, moral, medical, nursing, educational, social, and all other phases of hospital and nursing endeavor and other consistent purposes especially relating to the Catholic hospitals and schools of nursing in the United States and Canada."[93] Canada began its own separate health association in 1954, and the association in the United States became known as the Catholic Health Association of the United States (CHA). In 2004 the CHA provided strategic direction for sixty Catholic health care systems, including 617 hospitals with a presence in all fifty states.[94]

In 1921 the CHA wrote a small code of ethics that dealt with surgeries associated with pregnancy and reproduction. This code was replaced in 1949 by the first set of "Ethical and Religious Directives for Catholic Hospitals." These directives were originally meant to serve as guidelines for dioceses that did not have their own ethics codes.[95] The directives were revised in 1955, 1971, and most recently in 2001. They have become the standard and mandatory ethics code for all Catholic health care institutions in the United States. The directives are separated into an introduction and six chapters, or parts, dealing with a range of topics, from care at the beginning of life to care for the dying. They acknowledge that a right to adequate health care flows from human dignity and emphasize the "biblical mandate" requiring those in Catholic health care "to work to ensure that our country's health care delivery system provides adequate health care for the poor."[96]

In keeping with the spirit of the directives, since 1984 the CHA has written documents and formulated proposals to reform the United States' health care system. In 2000 it published its recommendations in a booklet titled *Continuing the Commitment: A Pathway to Health Care Reform*. The booklet begins with a description of the problems with the health care system in the United States, including the high numbers of uninsured and underinsured, the high and rising costs of health care, the growth in demand by patients, fragmented health care systems, problems with the financing of health care, and public apathy about the implications of the problems with the health care system.[97]

The booklet goes on to lay out what the CHA proposes to be foundational values for health care reform: the dignity of the person; the social nature of people; a duty to care for the poor and vulnerable; responsible stewardship; health care as an essential service, instead of a commodity; and health care that respects the religious and other ethical values of individuals and institutions.[98] Based on these values, the CHA developed eight guidelines for health care reform. First, health care must be universal, in that it should be available to all people regardless of employment, health status, or income. Second, a defined set of basic benefits should be available to all. Third, health care is a social good; therefore, it is a responsibility that should be shared by all members of society, along with government. Fourth, an appropriate use of resources consists of balancing the common good with individual needs and desires. Fifth, the financing of the health care system should be pluralistic, in that it should be shared between government, employers, and individuals, with progressive taxation as the preferred method of paying for the costs. Sixth, a high quality of health care based on compassion and respect should be promoted. Seventh, the participation of individuals to make choices about their health care should be encouraged. Finally, the CHA expressly acknowledged that changes to the health care system, although needed immediately, will be a gradual process.[99]

With these values and guidelines in mind, the CHA makes the following recommendations for health care reform. It begins by addressing private health insurance, calling for a system in which all people would be required to enroll in health plans. Moreover, it proposes that three levels of benefits should be available to meet the needs of all people; these health care plans should compete for consumer enrollment. To finance these plans, CHA advocates new federal initiatives to set minimum standards for benefits, establish premium subsidies, monitor changes in health insurance coverage and spending, and determine a way to pay for a "residual safety net–dependent population."[100] CHA also advocates an increase in Medicaid and Children's Health Insurance Program (CHIP) coverage, the establishment of a federal program to subsidize coverage for low- and middle-income people who cannot get employer-sponsored coverage, and a requirement that during an annual enrollment period, insurers cover all people without regard to preexisting conditions.[101]

The section on financing these recommendations is rather brief. The CHA suggests a "pluralistic" financing system, consisting of contributions from the federal government, employers, and individuals. It relies heavily on the federal and state governments to subsidize coverage for the elderly, the poor, and those with disabilities. The CHA does not provide any details on how much such a system might cost. It does acknowledge, however, that "additional public funding is almost certain to be required and should rely primarily on progressive rather than regressive funding mechanisms."[102]

The CHA makes a noble attempt to address health care reform. Yet, it does not address the most difficult funding questions. While advocating universal coverage, private insurance competition, and individual choice of insurance plans, it relies heavily on government oversight and funding but does not give many details regarding specific funding mechanisms, particularly market mechanisms. The plan, although strong on general values and guidelines, is weak on the specifics of costs and implementation.

The U.S. Catholic Bishops and Health Care

In 1981 the U.S. Catholic bishops issued their pastoral letter on health care. They begin by connecting health care and human dignity: "One's ability to live a fully human life and to reflect the unique dignity that belongs to each person is greatly affected by health."[103] They also acknowledge that health care is viewed by the Church as a basic human right that "flows from the sanctity of human life."[104]

Why is health care so important? They answer by looking at the ministry of Jesus and his acts of healing. Jesus emphasized the importance of healing and "demonstrated that illness could be an occasion to prove God's love for his people and not a sign of punishment."[105] The bishops suggest that in the biblical perspective health means wholeness. Biblical wholeness refers not just to the wholeness of the individual person but to the wholeness of society and its institutions, for it was Jesus who "proclaimed the kingdom of God on earth and reached out to touch and to heal our wounded humanity."[106] This healing ministry has continued in the Church ever since, not only through the sacramental ministry but also through health care services.

Out of respect for the unique dignity of beings created in the image of God, everyone is required to care for their own health as well as for the health of others. On a larger level, this means that society has an obligation to provide adequate health care. Since the "works of mercy" cannot be separated from the "works of justice," the bishops argue, Christians are required to "correct any unjust social, political and economic structures and institutions which are the causes of suffering."[107] Therefore, we all have a responsibility for health, a responsibility that lies at several levels. The individual is responsible to guard his or her own health, which includes reforming bad habits that adversely affect health. The family has an obligation to promote the health of its members through education and by setting good health examples. The Catholic parish should encourage its members in need of health care to use a Catholic hospital and to support local Catholic health care institutions. Parishioners should visit others from the parish who are ill or dying, and parishioners should advocate for the health needs of the poor. At the level of the diocese, church leaders should continue to advocate social and institutional changes that are needed to relieve economic conditions that contribute to poor health, such as inadequate housing and a polluted environment.[108]

The bishops also attempt to establish a "Catholic identity" regarding health care by suggesting that there are four major areas in which Catholic health care can distinguish itself from other health care institutions.[109] First, Catholic health care can offer personalized patient care amid the impersonal atmosphere of technology and medical science that permeates today's health care facilities. This can be done through strong pastoral care and chaplaincy departments. The second area in which Catholic health care can distinguish itself is through addressing the moral aspects of certain medical issues facing health care facilities. The bishops contend that *Ethical and Religious Directives for Catholic Health Care Services* identifies and resolves many such issues. For example, the directives expressly forbid abortion, contraceptive sterilization, and euthanasia. By offering guidelines on such issues, Catholic institutions provide firm standards to be followed that protect Catholic identity.

Another area in which Catholic health care distinguishes itself is its prophetic role. Catholic health care promotes Christian values, serving to fulfill the

Church's role as a prophetic voice. The bishops emphasize the Church's voice in helping the poor and vulnerable in society: "All those in the health apostolate who heed this call and follow the example of Jesus will continue to serve the poor, the frail elderly, the powerless and the alienated."[110] They advocate initiating programs on behalf of the poor by targeting rural and inner-city areas, where large proportions of the nation's poor live. They also promote the development of alternative models of health care, such as satellite clinics and home health care delivery.[111] The bishops further argue that Catholic health care can distinguish itself in the realm of employer-employee relations by allowing employees to organize and bargain collectively, receive just wages, and obtain just fringe benefits.

Finally, the bishops lay out some general principles for public health care policy. The first is that all people have a right to adequate health care regardless of their economic, social, or legal status. Second, any comprehensive health care system must be pluralistic, in that it should use public and private resources as well as the volunteer, religious, and other nonprofit sectors. Third, public policy should emphasize the promotion of health and prevention of disease. Fourth, the public should have a "reasonable" choice of health care providers, which may include individual or group providers, or even clinics or institutions. Fifth, uniform standards should be a part of the health care delivery system. Sixth, the bishops acknowledge that cost controls are necessary and call for such controls to be implemented at every level of health administration. Finally, the bishops call for the federal government to establish a comprehensive national health insurance program that is adequately funded and reflects "sound human values."[112] The bishops do not offer any specifics on how their vision of a health care system should be funded. Nor do they make any attempt to discuss the use of market mechanisms in the funding of health care.

The Catholic Medical Association

Beginning in 1912, guilds were established in cities in the eastern United States to provide spiritual retreats for Catholic physicians. By 1932 the National Federation of Catholic Physicians Guilds (NFCPG) was founded, and the publication *Linacre Quarterly* began. In 1944 the NFCPG became headquartered in St. Louis with what was still the Catholic Health Association of the United States and Canada.

In 1965 this relationship ended over a dispute about the funding and distribution of health care, with the CHA supporting strong government intervention.[113] In 1997 the board of directors of the NFCPG changed its name to the Catholic Medical Association (CMA). In May 2005 the CMA issued a statement on health care in America, reflecting a conservative tone, particularly when compared with its CHA counterpart. The CMA views the health care crisis in America as more than just a problem of lack of insurance. They see it as a crisis rooted in "the loss of a common understanding, within and without the medical profession, of the sanctity and inviolability of each human life."[114] The CMA is no fan of government. It is highly critical of government mandates requiring insurance coverage of contraceptives, sterilization, and genetic screening.[115]

The key to solving the health care crisis, according to the CMA, is to correct a crisis of "mis-insurance." One major reason for mis-insurance is that the right to health care has been misinterpreted. It has come to be understood as the individual patient's "radical autonomy, the triumph of relativism" to be enforced by the coercion of the state.[116] The CMA argues that the moral obligation to provide health care to others falls within the realm of charity, not within the dominion of justice and of governmental mandating of public policies to govern health care and insurance practices. It is not up to government or employers to fulfill this obligation. Rather, it is the responsibility of the individual and the family.[117]

To remedy the crisis of mis-insurance, the CMA recommends incentives in the form of refundable tax credits to enable people to buy their own insurance directly, instead of relying on employer-based insurance.[118] It also argues that insurance should be free from state and federal mandates because they drive up the costs of health care and restrict individual freedom of choice.[119] Finally, it advocates the use of health savings accounts, which are high-deductible insurance plans.[120]

The CMA's plan for health care reform lacks both substance and practicality, as seen in its promotion of high-deductible health plans. To use such accounts as well as benefit from tax incentives to purchase health plans, people must have a large amount of disposable income. Hence, they are out of reach for many Americans. I will analyze these accounts in more detail in the next chapter.

The CMA does not address other key problems associated with health insurance. For example, many chronically ill people are considered high risks and either cannot get coverage or cannot get it at a price they can afford. Furthermore, without some government regulation of insurance benefits, insurance policies become a mire of complicated and inconsistent provisions, leaving consumers somewhat confused and desperate in their attempts to discern what benefits are offered and guess which ones might be needed. The CMA's plan would simply widen the gap between those who can afford health care and those who cannot.

Conclusion: Justice, Capitalism, and Health Care

With its unique view of the person as created in the image of God, the Catholic justice tradition makes human dignity the starting place for assessing justice. Two important convictions of this tradition, grounded in the social nature of being human, are that people are interdependent and that the common good is more important than the good of the individual. Justice requires that we have a special obligation to the poor and vulnerable and that we be stewards over the resources of this earth. Moreover, the justice of any political, economic, or social institution must be interpreted from within the Christian framework of meaning, shaped by the life, teachings, Passion, death, and resurrection of Jesus Christ.

Hence, when assessing capitalism, the Church has often viewed it as morally limited. With its emphasis on profit, competition, and individualism, capitalism can threaten human dignity. Capitalism also often ignores the social purpose of private property and does not promote a healthy social interdependence among people. With its emphasis on individualism, capitalism encourages people to act out of personal self-interest rather than in the interest of the common good. In many countries with capitalistic economies, there are large disparities between the rich and poor, and the needs of the poor and vulnerable are easily overlooked. Capitalism also dismisses the importance of stewardship by ignoring the social dimension of private property. In fact, many of the values espoused by capitalism, such as profit, competition, and individualism, contradict such values found in Christianity as mercy, charity, and compassion.

The Church has deemed health care to be a basic right flowing from human dignity. Not only is some basic level of health required for all people to develop fully, but health care is viewed as a social good to serve the benefit of all in society. With its obligation to the poor and vulnerable, the Church also considers the just distribution of health care to be particularly important to those who suffer greatly because of their poverty. With a social justice tradition that finds capitalism morally limited, however, the Church faces a special challenge in trying to specify a method of justly distributing health care. Catholic social thought is vigorous in its support of universal health care, but it is relatively silent on the details of the distribution.

If capitalism is indeed an inherently unjust economic system, is its use an all-or-nothing affair? Or are there certain market mechanisms in the capitalistic system that can be used to fund and distribute health care and still meet the demands of Catholic social teaching on justice? To help answer these questions, the next chapter will explore health care economic theory.

Notes

1. Muller, *Mind and the Market*, xvi–xvii.
2. Plato, *Plato's Republic*, n. 550.
3. Viner, *Religious Thought and Economic Society*, 35.
4. Ibid., 35–36.
5. Muller, *Mind and the Market*, 7.
6. Groethuysen, *The Bourgeois*, 191–92.
7. For an excellent discussion on the history of the Church's position on usury, see Jonsen and Toulmin, *Abuse of Casuistry*, 181–94.
8. Muller, *Mind and the Market*, 11.
9. Leo XIII, *Rerum novarum*, n. 2.
10. Muller, *Mind and the Market*, 12.
11. Ibid., 51.
12. Adam Smith, *Wealth of Nations*, 70.
13. Ibid., 67.
14. Ibid., 68.
15. Ibid., 146.
16. Muller, *Mind and the Market*, xvii.
17. Ibid., 61.
18. Yergin and Stanislaw, *Commanding Heights*, 353–67.
19. United States Catholic Conference, *Catechism of the Catholic Church*, n. 2425.
20. Massaro, *Living Justice*, 176–77.
21. U.S. Catholic Bishops, "Economic Justice for All," n. 13.
22. Leo XIII, *Rerum novarum*, nos. 31–38.
23. Pius XI, *Quadragesimo anno*, nos. 47–49.
24. John XXIII, *Mater et magistra*, n. 82.
25. John XXIII, *Pacem in terris*, nos. 18–20.
26. Paul VI, *Popularum progressio*, n. 26.
27. Paul VI, *Octogesima adveniens*, n. 35.

28. John Paul II, *Laborem exercens,* n. 3.

29. Ibid., n. 7.

30. Ibid., n. 13.

31. Ibid.

32. Ibid., n. 14.

33. Ibid.

34. John Paul II, *Sollicitudo rei socialis,* n. 42.

35. Ibid., n. 37.

36. Ibid.

37. John Paul II, *Centesimus annus,* n. 42.

38. Ibid., n. 4.

39. Ibid., n. 6.

40. Ibid., n. 8.

41. Ibid., n. 10.

42. Ibid., n. 36.

43. Ibid., n. 32.

44. Ibid., n. 42.

45. Ibid., n. 15.

46. Ibid.

47. Ibid., n. 34.

48. Ryan wrote several important books on economic policy, including *Living Wage* and *Distributive Justice.*

49. Administration Board, *Our Bishops Speak,* 243–60.

50. The library at the Catholic University of America contains a large collection of archives from the NCWC.

51. Administration Board, *Our Bishops Speak,* 298.

52. Dolan, "Bishops in Council," 22.

53. U.S. Catholic Bishops, "Economic Justice for All," n. 12.

54. Ibid., n. 13–18.

55. Ibid., n. 132.

56. Ibid., n. 115.

57. Ibid., nos. 90a–90d.

58. Ibid., n. 102–215.

59. Novak, *Spirit of Democratic Capitalism,* 182–86.

60. Ibid., 14.

61. Novak, *Toward a Theology of the Corporation,* 8.

62. Novak, "Good Capitalist," 30.

63. Ibid.

64. Ibid.

65. Novak, "Seven Theological Facets," 117–18.

66. Levinson and de Onis, *Alliance That Lost Its Way*, 8–16.

67. For an excellent resource, see Christian Smith, *The Emergence of Liberation Theology*.

68. Segundo, *Liberation of Theology*, 8.

69. Latin American Bishops Conference, "Medillín Documents: Peace," 455.

70. Latin American Bishops Conference, "Medellín Documents: Justice," 449.

71. Bonino, *Doing Theology in a Revolutionary Situation*, 31.

72. Gutiérrez, *Theology of Liberation*, 66.

73. John Paul II, "The Pope at Puebla," 62.

74. Smith, *Emergence of Liberation Theology*, 224–25.

75. Fraser and Jeffrey, "Poverty Cuts Children's Chances," 13.

76. Ibid., 13–14.

77. Hollenbach, *Common Good and Christian Ethics*, 184.

78. Ibid.

79. U.S. Census Bureau, "Income, Poverty and Health Insurance Coverage." The poverty level was set at $19,484 for a family of four.

80. Fraser and Jeffrey, "Call for Economic Change," 19.

81. Ibid.

82. David F. Kelly, *Emergence of Roman Catholic Medical Ethics*, 24.

83. Ibid., 30–31.

84. Ibid., 31–37.

85. For an overview of the history of pastoral medicine, see ibid., 44–81.

86. Ibid., 47.

87. Ibid., 48.

88. Ibid., 48–49.

89. Ibid., 50–51.

90. Ibid., 161–62.

91. For a more detailed description of these works, see Ibid., 181–219.

92. John XXIII, *Pacem in terris*, n. 11.

93. *New Catholic Encyclopedia*, 1st ed., s.v. "Catholic Hospital Association."

94. Catholic Health Association of the United States, *Catholic Health Care*, 2.

95. Kelly, *Emergence of Roman Catholic Medical Ethics*, 173.

96. National Conference of Catholic Bishops, *Ethical and Religious Directives*, pt. 1, introduction.

97. Catholic Health Association of the United States, *Continuing the Commitment*, 1–5.

98. Ibid., 7.

99. Ibid., 8–9.

100. Ibid., 12.

101. Ibid., 11–12.

102. Ibid., 13.

103. National Conference of Catholic Bishops, "U.S. Bishops' Pastoral Letter," 397.

104. Ibid.

105. Ibid.

106. Ibid.

107. Ibid., 398.

108. Ibid., 398–99.

109. Ibid., 400–402.

110. Ibid., 400.

111. Ibid., 401.

112. Ibid., 402.

113. Bissonnette-Pitre, "Brief History."

114. Catholic Medical Association, "Health Care in America," 93.

115. Ibid., 93–96.

116. Ibid., 104.

117. Ibid., 106.

118. Ibid., 106–7.

119. Ibid., 108.

120. Ibid., 109–10.

CHAPTER 3

Health Care Economic Theory, Market Mechanisms, and Health Outcomes

We now move from Catholic social thought to secular health care economics. There are two distinct layers of controversy within this arena. The first is the theoretical debate, where the focus is on whether various economic theories are compatible with, or even apply to, the field of health care. Some economists argue health care is so different from other enterprises that certain economic theories simply do not apply. The second layer of debate is on actual market practices and how they affect specific health outcomes. I will explore each of these dimensions after discussing the history of market mechanism use in health care.

When beginning to discuss market theory and health care, it is important to clarify the term *market*, specifically in relation to its use in a health care setting. Traditionally, a market is seen as a system of exchange of wages and goods based on supply and demand and not regulated by government.[1] When the term is used in relation to health care, though, the standard definition is not suitable. There is no nation with a purely market-run health care system or with a purely government-run one. Rather, there are various combinations of government and market controls.

In health care economics the major debate centers on the use of certain market-style incentives, mechanisms whose purpose generally is to influence profit. Incentives can also be used within a nonprofit institution, however, to influence the behavior of doctors or patients, the goal being that the institution remain financially solvent. Mark Peterson summarizes market mechanisms as follows: "They often refer to the use of incentives embedded within institutions of whatever sort (private or public) that are designed to encourage more efficient individual-level behavior."[2]

A Short History of Medicine and the Market

Apparently, there were no market characteristics in medicine until the end of the eighteenth century. Prior to that there was no real competition for patients among doctors. Medicine could not cure or treat many diseases or injuries. In fact, doctors often actually accidentally killed their patients. There was no real competition for the services of doctors, and medicine was not viewed as "a necessity of life," as it is today.[3]

In their 2006 book *Medicine and the Market: Equity v. Choice*, Daniel Callahan and Angela Wasunna explore the question, How did medicine eventually come to be seen as a profitable commodity? They conclude that four factors contributed to the change in the social and economic status of medicine. The first is what they call "a new vision of medical possibilities," stemming from the Enlightenment hope that through science, anything was possible. Optimism that all diseases could eventually be prevented or cured has flourished since then.

This theme has been particularly strong in the United States, where in 1914 a doctor wrote in the *Journal of the American Medical Association* that "in fifty years science will have practically eliminated all forms of disease."[4] By the mid-twentieth century, the National Institutes of Health (NIH), the national medical and behavioral institute, was thriving. It was given bureau status in 1943 and continued to expand over the next several decades. National commitments have been made to end various diseases; for example, in 1970 President Richard Nixon declared a war on cancer.

In 1990 an international consortium of scientists united to map the entire human genome systematically, in what became known as the Human Genome Project. Eventually, rivalry developed when a private U.S. corporation took on the same challenge. In 2000 the consortium and the private scientists jointly announced that their researchers, working separately, had sequenced the genome. Substantial rhetoric about the potential that this project may have on the prevention and curing of major diseases followed the completion of the sequencing.[5]

Today a national debate over using embryonic stem cells in research is ongoing. Some scientists claim that embryonic stem cells have the potential to treat or even cure several horrible diseases and afflictions, such as diabetes, Parkinson's disease, and spinal cord injuries. Other scientists point out that despite the enormous amount of money being spent on embryonic stem cell research, it has resulted in little or no success in treating medical conditions.

Another factor contributing to the change in the status of medicine in recent centuries was a decline in mortality and morbidity. Callahan and Wasunna point out that since the year 1800, when the average person lived to be thirty-five years old, average life expectancy has increased markedly. In 2001 the average life expectancy for the total population in the United States was 77.2 years; in 1900 it was 47.3 years.[6] In 1915 the average infant mortality rate was 100 infant deaths per 1000 births for white babies and almost twice that rate for black babies; in 2001 the average was only 6.9 infant deaths per 1000 live births.[7]

Many factors can be given to help account for this phenomenon. A United Nations study cites the occurrence of better living conditions, exemplified by improved nutrition and housing; major public sanitation projects; and after 1900 a combination of medical, economic, and public health developments.[8] Moreover, there has been a shift in the type of diseases that are prevalent in developed countries, from the communicable diseases that were dominant prior to 1900, such as smallpox, diphtheria, and scarlet fever, to the noncommunicable diseases of today, such as heart and respiratory diseases as well as cancer.[9]

Callahan and Wasunna argue that a third factor contributing to a major change in the social and economic status of medicine is an acceptance of medical research. By the end of the nineteenth century, medical schools and the pharmaceutical industry had organized efforts to promote research. Formal efforts began in Germany, where universities and medical schools received governmental support to do major medical research.

Germany served as a model for the United States, where research became an integral part of medical schools and became associated with their prestige. Private philanthropic funding of medical research also took off. In 1901 John D. Rockefeller established the nation's first independent research institute, the Rockefeller Institute for Medical Research, which later became the Rockefeller University.[10]

Drug development and the pharmaceutical industry in the United States have fascinating histories.[11] Early medicinal remedies included roots, berries, leaves, and bark. In the early nineteenth century, medicines for ailments such as headaches, constipation, and coughs were widely advertised. These medicines were not regulated by law and often contained alcohol or opiates, which were not disclosed to the consumer. The Pure Food and Drug Act was enacted as a response in 1906, eventually leading to the establishment of the Food and Drug Administration in 1930.

In *What Price Better Health? Hazards of the Research Imperative*, Daniel Callahan names three major developments in the pharmaceutical industry in the nineteenth century: Alkaloid chemistry was used to extract compounds from plants; synthetic dyes were developed from coal tar; and drug research was formalized.[12] By the late nineteenth century and early twentieth century, drug research was making rapid gains. Antibiotics, such as streptomycin and penicillin, were developed. In the 1970s new drugs were developed in response to the rapidly increasing knowledge of the molecular biology of the human organism. By the 1990s this type of drug research had become popular, giving birth to the whole biotechnology industry and biotech companies, such as Genentech and Amgen.[13]

The pharmaceutical industry has since become the most lucrative industry in the United States. In 2005 total international sales of pharmaceuticals in ten key countries were $602 billion. This figure represents a 5.7 percent growth rate over the previous year. North America alone accounted for $265.7 billion in retail pharmaceutical sales.[14]

The United States government has also become heavily involved with medical research, as evidenced by the expansion of the NIH. Originally funded as a small research effort of the federal government in 1879, it has grown into a massive organization consisting of twenty-seven separate institutes and centers—devoted to research on a variety of diseases, illnesses, and conditions, ranging from cancer to gerontology to drug abuse—with a budget of over $23 billion. It is one of eight health agencies of the Public Health Service, which is part of the United States Department of Health and Human Services.

Callahan and Wasunna's final factor contributing to the change in the status of medicine is the reemergence of a medical market. In the nineteenth and early twentieth centuries, there had been a small but disenfranchised market. At the beginning of the twentieth century, there were 162 medical schools, many of them for-profit. In 1910 for-profit hospitals constituted about 56 percent of the total number of hospitals in the United States. By 1946, though, for-profit hospitals accounted for only 18 percent.[15] Managing a hospital for a profit was generally not considered a good idea. Indeed, the American Medical Association had stated in 1929 that doctors who tried to make a profit by running hospitals discovered the hospital to be "a losing proposition."[16] Also, proprietary medical schools had a hard time staying in the black, for many reasons, and by the early twentieth century, most had fallen by the wayside.[17]

So, exactly when did medicine look to the market as a way to manage and organize health care? There are many theories purporting to provide answers to this question, but there does not seem to be any specific time that this occurred. Rather, as Callahan speculates, it appears that it was government's involvement in health care that opened the door for market mechanisms. According to Paul Starr, whose book *The Social Transformation of American Medicine* details the history of American medicine, the onset of World War II, even more than the New Deal, led to a large expansion of the federal government's financial support of medicine. Since before World War I, most funding for medical research came from private sources.[18] However, research became a priority with the onset of World War II. In July 1942 President Roosevelt established the Office of Scientific Research and Development (OSRD), which consisted of two committees, one on national defense and the other on medical research. The Committee on Medical Research (CMR) supported research on war-related medical problems. One such problem was malaria. The Japanese had taken control of the sources for quinine in the Pacific, so a synthetic source was needed. Researchers under contract with the CMR developed quinacrine (Atabrine), which was more effective than quinine in the treatment of malaria.[19] Researchers also improved the strains of, and method for producing, penicillin.[20]

Interest in public health care also grew. The NIH saw a tremendous expansion in the 1940s, its budget going from $180 thousand in 1945 to $4 million in 1947.[21] Large hospital expansion programs were started, in part to create jobs under New Deal public works programs. Also, a large number of returning war veterans would need medical assistance. So, right after the end of the war, two major hospital construction programs were initiated. One federal bill funded new Veterans Administration hospitals and encouraged their affiliation with medical schools.[22] A second bill, known as the Hill–Burton Act, provided construction money for community hospitals.[23] This infusion of money into research, hospitals, and training spurred more growth in the medical industry. The decade of the 1950s saw tremendous growth in the number of medical schools, medical interns and residents, and medical specialties.[24]

The 1960s were a time of immense change and reform in the United States. Many federally funded programs were developed to help the poor, including Head Start, Volunteers in Service to America (Vista), and Legal Services for the Poor. This same trend was seen in health care. The Kerr–Mills Act in 1960 provided large matching federal grants to states to encourage them to develop health care programs for the elderly poor and nonelderly disabled. The program was criticized by many senior citizens groups, though, because the funds were not distributed evenly, with much of the money going to a small number of states.[25]

In November 1964 Lyndon Johnson, running for president on a platform of "Great Society" reforms, won a landslide victory over Barry Goldwater. The next year Congress passed, and Johnson signed into law, the Medicare program for the elderly and the Medicaid program for the poor. Today the Medicare program consists of two parts. Part A provides a hospital insurance program for people over the age of sixty-five who have social security benefits. Part A is mandatory and is financed by a special social security tax paid by all workers. Part B is a voluntary plan that provides coverage for doctors and other medical services. It is paid for by beneficiary premiums and contributions from the U.S. Treasury. It is important to note that Medicare is both a contributory program as well as an entitlement program. It is contributory in that all people who work pay into the program through a tax on their earnings. It is an entitlement program due to the fact that everyone is eligible for Medicare upon reaching the age of sixty-five, or if they are younger and meet certain disability requirements.

The Medicaid program provides assistance to poor people who are eligible for state-run welfare programs. It is administered by the states under federal guidelines that require that specific minimum standards of coverage be met. Medicaid is funded by both the federal government and state governments. It is a public-assistance, or welfare, program in which people must qualify in order to receive benefits. It is also an entitlement program because all people who meet the qualifications are entitled to receive Medicaid.

Throughout the ensuing years after the passage of Medicare and Medicaid, medical costs rose sharply, with government's share of costs rapidly increasing, as well. In the seven years before the creation of Medicare, the inflation rate of medical costs was 3.2 percent a year; in the five following years, it rose to average 7.9 percent per year.[26] Between 1960 and 1965, per capita health expenditures went from $142 to $198. By 1970 per capita costs were at $336.[27] The impact of medical costs on the federal government was immense. Between 1965 and 1970, the government's share of health expenditures rose from 26 to 37 percent. The government spent $10.8 billion in health expenditures in 1965; by 1970 it spent $27.8 billion.[28]

Rising health care costs became a hot political issue. In 1971, in order to attempt to control costs, President Richard Nixon's administration promoted and won backing for a "health maintenance strategy" that supported and subsidized health maintenance organizations, which later became known as HMOs.[29] HMOs brought a multitude of problems into the realm of health care. By the time President Bill Clinton took office in 1993, many felt the health care system needed a major overhaul. In an effort to create a universal health care system, Clinton proposed the Clinton Health Security Bill, legislation that would cover everyone in the United States while embodying the key market concept of competition. His bill was originally based on the "managed competition" theory of Stanford professor Alain Enthoven, whose ideas will be examined in detail in the next chapter. By the time Enthoven's theories were put into legislative form, they had been watered down considerably. Regardless, the Clinton health care proposal failed, for many reasons, leaving the United States with a costly health care system that covered fewer and fewer people.

In response to the failed attempt to get universal health care in the United States, many health care advocates focused on expanding coverage for children. In 1997 Congress passed the State Children's Health Insurance Program (SCHIP), which provides funds to the individual states to expand health insurance coverage to children who are uninsured or from low-income or moderate-income families.

The trends of rising health care costs and a rising number of uninsured people continue. In 2002 health care spending in the United States hit an all-time high of $1.6 trillion, which was a 9.3 percent increase over just the previous year. Government spent $713.4 billion for health care in 2002.[30] In fact, health care spending amounts to 14.9 percent of the gross domestic product (GDP) in the United States, which is a higher percentage than any other country in the world.[31] The trend continued. In 2004, 15 per cent of the GDP was spent on health care.[32] Yet, even with these large expenditures on health care, in 2004 there were still 45.5 million Americans without any type of health insurance.[33] With a record that has resulted in at best mixed results, many see the decades of government involvement in health care as proof that government should not be involved in the organization and financing of health care.

Given this perceived failure on the part of government and the undeniability of continually rising costs of health care and more uninsured people, market proponents are trying to make their case. Although the reasons for this situation have always been hotly debated, market proponents suggest that competition among health care providers and fewer government regulations would control costs and make the health care system more efficient.

Politically, market proponents have made inroads. President Bush is a market proponent, and he has called for the privatization of the Medicare program.

A good example of the debate over privatization was the Medicare drug benefit proposal of 2003. This debate appeared to center on the question of expanding Medicare benefits to include prescription drugs. In reality, the debate went much deeper. The real fight was over ideology. On one side were the market proponents, who, according to the *Wall Street Journal's* coverage of the Medicare debate, want "to widen the role of private health plans and force government-run Medicare to compete directly with the private alternatives. The only way to make Medicare affordable in the long run, conservatives contend, is to rely more on the market."[34] On the other side of the debate were congressional Democrats, who argued that "only by safeguarding the traditional government program . . . can the government ensure that all elderly, regardless of income, continue to get health care."[35] In the end a prescription drug plan passed the Congress. With a budget of $400 billion, the new legislation contains several market features, including health savings accounts, subsidies to support private health plans that compete with Medicare, a 28 percent tax exemption for corporations that give retirees drug benefits, and the use of private insurance companies to help manage the new plan.

Traditional Market Economic Theory

To evaluate when market practices in health care would and would not be consistent with Catholic social teaching, and to make some recommendation about the possibilities and limits of market practices in health care, it is important to review some of the major economic issues. Health care economics is a large, multifaceted subject. It is my intention to give the reader merely an overview of some of the major areas of contention among health care economists.

The main question among health care economists is this: Is the health care sector so different that it cannot be governed by the market like other sectors? We will first look at two economists who argue that it is. Then we will look at an essay by two economists who argue that although traditional market theory has some flaws, it can and should apply to health care. Before exploring these views, it is important first to understand the main tenets of traditional market theory.

Theory of Competition

In a competitive market there are two basic groups of players: *consumers*, who have money to exchange for goods; and *producers*, who have goods or services to exchange for money. The amount of a good or service that consumers would like to purchase at a particular time is called the *demand* for that good or service. The amount of the good or service that producers would like to sell is called the *supply* of the good or service.

In *consumer theory* there is an assumption that people seek to maximize the *utility* derived from purchasing goods and services, resulting in happiness. Jeremy Bentham (1748–1832), the father of utilitarianism, proposed the principle of utility, that is, that individuals should act in such a way that results in the greatest happiness of all those in question. He formulated a mathematical pleasure-over-pain ratio to apply to every individual who would be affected by a law or policy. Bentham argued that an action is right as long as it tends to increase the sum total of pleasure or diminish the sum total of pain.[36]

Utilitarianism has evolved, and today some economists disregard the theory entirely, anyway. Still, there are two key utilitarianism assumptions important to our purposes: Utility can be quantified, and it can be derived for a population by adding the utility "scores" of multiple individuals (known as *cardinal utility*). Modern economists have generally rejected Bentham's notion of cardinal utility and replaced it with the concept of *ordinal utility*, which holds that an individual simply chooses the bundle of goods (the aggregate of purchases) that he or she prefers, without quantifying how much utility is derived from one bundle over another.[37] Each individual has his or her own ideal bundle of goods and services that he or she wants to possess, which is determined by the desirability of each good or service, the prices of competing goods and services, and the amount of money available to spend on goods and services. The consumer maximizes utility by spending every successive dollar in such a manner that brings him or her the most happiness. The underlying premise in consumer theory thus boils down to the notion that people have the ability to make the best choices for themselves by following their own preferences and taking into account market prices.[38]

In *production theory* firms are thought to maximize profits much like consumers are thought to maximize utility. They are motivated primarily by their drive to make profit. In order to maximize profits, producers must buy certain inputs and then use some type of technology to turn the inputs into certain outputs. The number of inputs purchased depends on what is needed for each output and how much each input costs. In order to maximize profits, production firms must use inputs that cost the least. This behavior is supposed to result in societal benefits by not wasting inputs and by producing only the goods and services that consumers demand.[39]

When consumer and producer markets are in equilibrium and consumers' relative desire for either of a pair of goods is equal to the economy's ability to transform one good into the other (they are economically interchangeable), the economy is said to be in a Pareto optimal state. The Pareto principle holds that "if every member of a society prefers one alternative, say A, to another alternative, say B, then A is better than B. . . . A choice is said to be *Pareto optimal* if there is no other choice which would be preferred to it under the Pareto principle."[40] In other words, if certain conditions are met, market competition on its own will cause a situation where one cannot make someone better off without making someone else worse off. Pareto optimality is, therefore, a criterion used to assess forms of economic organization.

Demand Theory

Demand for goods and services drives the market economy. In *demand theory* the amount of a particular good or service that is produced and consumed is determined by the amount of demand for it. Demand is reflected in "how many goods and services are purchased at alternative prices."[41] If, for some reason, the demand for a specific item changes (decreases) because people decide they want a different product, the price of the first item will change (will drop), and the producer will adjust its production accordingly (making less of the item). Over time the supply of the increasingly popular item will be adjusted (will increase) to satisfy demand, unless there is some shortage of a particular input for production (such as a raw material or skilled labor).[42]

How can demand be determined? Rice points out that one method is simply to ask a person which bundle of goods, among alternatives, he or she prefers. Of course, it would be difficult to survey an entire population. Moreover, people may not tell the truth.[43] So, economist Paul Samuelson created an economic concept known as *revealed preference*, which assumes that people must "prefer" whatever bundle of goods they choose. If people choose certain bundles of goods over alternative affordable bundles, "they have revealed themselves to prefer the former."[44] It is implied that the specific goods and services that people demand are the ones that make them best off, all factors considered.

The revealed preference theory also implies that the utility derived from purchasing a particular good or service is at least as great as the price paid for it, or the consumer would not have bought it to begin with. A demand curve reveals a specific purchase's *marginal utility*, the change in total satisfaction as a result of consuming one additional unit of a specific good or service. For example, if someone is willing to buy five loaves of bread at $1.00 per loaf but then buys six loaves of bread at 80 cents per loaf, the marginal utility derived from the purchase of the sixth loaf of bread is at least 80 cents. Since people are thought to always maximize their utility, it is theorized that they will buy only goods whose marginal utilities equal or surpass the market prices.

Consumer surplus is a related concept. When a consumer buys a good that costs less than the maximum amount he or she would have been willing to pay, the difference is consumer surplus. At the aggregate level, adding together all of the surpluses "received" by all consumers, total consumer surplus is the difference between the value consumers receive from goods and how much they have to pay for them.[45] The concept of aggregate consumer surplus is used by economists to ascertain, for example, whether a publicly financed project should go forward. It is hoped that the project's value to the whole community or society, minus the total costs (as borne by taxes and so on), would result in an overall surplus.

Supply Theory

Supply theory is another major ingredient in *microeconomics*, the branch of economics that studies individual consumers, households, and firms. *Supply* is defined as the quantity of a good that sellers would like to sell during a certain period and at a certain price.[46] The point at which supply and demand intersect, or are equal, indicates the price of the goods or services to be exchanged as well as the amount of goods and services exchanged. The market is said to be in equilibrium when supply and demand are equal and the desires of those exchanging goods or services are mutually consistent. At equilibrium prices people can buy or sell all that they want within their budgets.[47] If a price is higher than the equilibrium price, then supply will be greater than demand. This is called *excess supply*. If the opposite occurs, then demand will be greater than supply, a situation known as *excess demand*.[48]

In order to understand the relation between supply and profits, it is important to recognize that total costs are divided into variable and fixed costs. *Variable costs* change with the amount of output. *Fixed costs* do not change. Examples of fixed costs are land and capital purchases. A *supply curve* is an upward-sloping curve showing the relationship between price and the amount of a good or service supplied by a seller. The higher the prices are for a particular good or service, the greater the supply the seller would like to have, in order to make more profit per sale. The converse is also true: The lower the price for that same item, the lower the supply the seller would want to have, because profit would be lower per sale.[49]

Two major factors cause supply curves to shift. A change in the cost of the inputs used to produce a good or service will decrease profits and make production less attractive, resulting in reduced supply. Second, a new technological breakthrough can reduce production costs and therefore increase profits, likely resulting in greater supply.[50]

According to Thomas Rice, in most uses of economic theory, supply plays a subsidiary role to demand. The reason is that if demand for a particular good or service declines, producers will usually produce less of the product. The opposite is true as well: If demand increases, producers will produce more of the product, or more producers will enter the market to sell the product.

Rice argues that health care is different from most other industries. In health care, supply plays a major role in determining both prices and output.

Income Distribution

Income distribution is one of the most controversial issues in economic theory. Income is unequally distributed in the United States. As pointed out in the last chapter, over 12 percent of people in the United States live at or below the poverty level. In traditional microeconomics, issues concerning the equitability of the distribution of wealth are often ignored. Proponents of market economics argue that through competition, resources are distributed in such a manner that reflects the desires of society. Income is usually distributed in the form of wages (salaries, all labor income, commissions) and profits.[51] Market proponents justify the uneven distribution of income by arguing that wages and profits are earned by the sacrifices and productivity of capitalists, and, therefore, whatever the resulting income distribution is, it is just and equitable.[52] Traditional economics rests on the theory that competition is positive and that the results of this competition, whatever they may be, are, in general, socially desirable.

Yet government has a role altering the distribution of resources among the general population.

The Role of Government

An essential question in market economics is what role, if any, government should play. Traditional economic theory encourages government involvement to overcome market failures that cause inefficient outcomes or uneven distribution of resources. The government does this in many ways, including overseeing the quality of consumer products, monitoring consumer information to ensure its accuracy, and enacting antitrust legislation.

Thomas Rice groups the types of possible market failures into four categories. Sometimes certain *structural deficiencies* exist in a market. Insufficient consumer information is one such deficiency. Market economic theory relies heavily on the concept that consumers maximize their utility through making choices about desired goods or services. Without sufficient information about the various alternatives, it is impossible for consumers to make utility-maximizing choices.[53] Another type of structural deficiency occurs when a producer has a monopoly on a product or service. If no alternative exists, then the consumer is not making a choice at all. A firm charging too high a price in a competitive market would lower demand; with a monopoly it can raise a price without losing its whole market.[54]

A second type of market failure requiring government involvement concerns when the product in question is a *public good*, which Rice defines as "one in which the consumption by one person does not diminish its consumption by another; a second characteristic is that it is nearly impossible to exclude someone from using the good."[55] Public goods are rarely produced by the market, because it is difficult to make profits off them. When the market fails to provide a given public good that is somehow considered necessary, or at least desirable, it may have to be up to government to use tax revenue to finance it. National defense and clean air are examples of public goods. However, just because something is a public good, it does not mean that government automatically should be involved in its production or provision. Costs and overall gain to society must first be considered.[56]

A third type of market failure warranting government involvement is where *externalities* are associated with a product or service. A consumption externality exists "when one person's consumption of a good or service has an effect on the utility of another person."[57] A positive externality raises the utility of the other, whereas a negative externality lowers it. Government may step in to promote a positive externality or suppress a negative externality when the market can't or won't.

As an example of a negative externality, Rice mentions that cigarette and cigar smoking in a public place may negatively affect the health of nonsmokers there. Governments, often municipalities and even states have enacted ordinances and legislation banning smoking in certain public places because the benefit to the public is considered very strong.

Immunizations are an example of a positive externality because when one individual gets an immunization against a given disease, this makes it statistically less likely that a nonimmunized person will get the disease. In a competitive market many individuals would probably not want to pay for the immunization. In such a case it may be better if the government subsidizes or outright pays for the immunizations because the benefits for the whole society are so great.[58]

Another type of market failure calling for government involvement is where a product or service is characterized by *increasing returns to scale*. Usually, when a producer broadens the use of inputs by a certain amount, the corresponding increase in output is either the same or less than the increase in input. Known as constant or decreasing returns to scale, this condition implies that there is no advantage in having a monopoly. If there were increasing returns to scale, the average cost of production would decrease, as the number of producers that supply part of the output declines until just one producer supplies all of the output.[59] If this were the case, then monopolies might actually benefit society. As noted earlier, though, in a competitive market monopolies are believed to stifle choice, price competition, and efficiency.

Under traditional market theory, if any of these four market failures occurs—there is a structural deficiency in a market, a product or service is a public good that the market is not motivated to supply, the product or service has an externality that the market is not motivated to deal with, or the product or service is characterized by increasing returns to scale—government may be able to intervene and provide greater efficiency and utility than the market. Government could fail to do a better job than the market, though. There is not much economics literature on government failure at intervention. Charles Wolf, a pioneer in the field of government failure, argues that intervention presents unique challenges. The government is basically a monopoly and does not have the same budget constraints that other businesses do. Whereas most businesses must stick to a strict bottom line regarding profits and losses, government does not. Many of the products that private businesses sell can be defined, and their output measured, easily; with many government programs, such as public education, it is difficult to measure outcomes. Government is also run by politicians, who can be shortsighted and who can abruptly be voted out of office.[60]

Other economists have come up with theories arguing that government regulations do not serve the public but rather serve the people that they are supposed to regulate. For example, regulations that restrict competitors or make entry into a market difficult (such as professional licensing) can be viewed as anticompetition and inefficient. Moreover, politicians themselves as well as their staffs have vested interests in keeping their jobs. Hence, some economists theorize, they may cater to special interest groups as a means of survival.[61]

Health Care Economics: The Debate

The first part of this chapter summarized the main tenets of traditional market economic theory. Now I shall address the question raised at the beginning of this chapter: Does market economic theory apply to the realm of health care, or is providing health care so different from providing other goods and services that market theory does not apply? There is an abundance of literature on this subject, and I shall review some of the major arguments in this debate, beginning with the view that many assumptions of market theory simply do not apply to health care.

The Naysayers

In 1963 Stanford economist Kenneth Arrow wrote an article for the *American Economic Review* arguing that the "medical-care industry" is not a good candidate for the market.[62] His article has since become a classic and is often referenced in health care economic literature. It spawned a good deal of discussion about market failures and health care markets.[63] Arrow begins his argument by noting that the medical-care industry has special economic problems that separate it from the economic "norm," the traditional competitive model.[64] The first special problem is the characteristics of a person's demand for medical services. It is not steady, as is the demand for other goods, such as food or clothing. Instead, except for preventative services, satisfaction of the demand for health care is obtained only if there is an illness. Arrow suggests that this fact makes health care unique.

Medical problems, in addition to being quite expensive, Arrow argues, also place a particularly heavy burden on the individual patient (consumer). There is often a chance that the individual might lose his or her earning ability, or even a chance of death or disability.[65]

Another reason medical services differ from the traditional competitive model is their uniqueness as a commodity. Arrow suggests that health care is a type of commodity where the product and the activity of the production are the same. The consumer is not able to test the product before purchasing it. Moreover, the uncertain quality of the health care product—patient health—is intense, because recovery from an illness or other medical condition can be very unpredictable.

There is also an important element of trust in the patient-physician relationship. The physician is therefore expected to behave in a manner different from that of sellers or producers of other goods or services. Arrow gives several examples to illustrate his point. A physician is supposed to give advice that is separated from his or her own self-interest. The treatment prescribed is supposed to be based on the objective needs of the patient and not influenced by the patient's financial considerations. A physician is also seen as an expert in certifying the existence of illnesses and injuries for legal and other purposes. Thus, the physician's concern for making correct diagnoses may outweigh his or her desire to please the patient.[66] These behaviors affect profit motive. Arrow claims that it is for these reasons that there is a prevalence of nonprofit entities in the field of health care.[67] Moreover, because medicine is a complicated field, the physician knows a lot more than the average patient. Arrow acknowledges that there is almost always some discrepancy between the information possessed by a producer and that by a consumer, but, he contends, this discrepancy is much more pronounced in health care.[68]

Yet another major difference is that the supply of most commodities is governed by the net return from production, compared with the return derived from the use of the same resources elsewhere.[69] Arrow argues that the health care industry is an exception. For one thing, the medical profession requires licensing, which restricts the supply and increases the costs.[70] Second, the cost of a medical education is very high and is often not paid for by the student him- or herself. Hence, the student's personal benefit outweighs the costs, creating a sort of subsidy, which, in theory, should cause the price of medical services to fall. Yet, the subsidies are offset by a restriction on entrance into medical schools and by the elimination of some students from medical school. Arrow claims that the practices of restricting entry to subsidized education and requiring licenses limit the possibility of alternative avenues in medical care, so both the quantity and quality of medical care are being influenced by nonmarket forces.[71]

Arrow concludes his essay this way: "The failure of the market to insure against uncertainties has created many social institutions in which the usual assumptions of the market are to some extent contradicted. The medical profession is only one example, though in many respects an extreme case."[72]

Thomas Rice, who has already been mentioned in connection with economic theory, contends that many of the assumptions raised in traditional market theory simply cannot be met in the health care sector. In the second edition of his book *The Economics of Health Reconsidered*, he discusses in detail what he claims to be numerous assumptions that simply do not apply to health care.

The first inapplicable assumption is that there are no externalities of consumption. Rice argues that in order for market competition to be superior to other economic systems, there cannot be any externalities of consumption, or if there are any, they must be dealt with through public policy that either taxes or subsidizes the good or service.[73] If certain externalities exist, then market competition will not result in a socially optimal outcome.

Rice contends that both negative and positive externalities of consumption do exist. He argues that a person's concern about status creates a negative externality. He contends that economic theory should not ignore how one person's bundle of goods and services compares with and affects, or is affected by, the bundles that other people have.[74] Traditional market theory does not consider that people are concerned about their status in society, but Rice says people do care about what others around them possess. If people have strong positive or negative feelings about what others around them possess, then a competitive market may not be best for the overall welfare of society. To illustrate his point, Rice uses the example of purchasing an automobile. If your neighbor makes you unhappy by buying a fancy car, the societal marginal utility (the overall benefit to all concerned) from that purchase will be lower than your neighbor's personal marginal utility.

The second externality, the positive one, is the fact that people in general care about the well-being of others.[75] To illustrate this, Rice uses the example of concern for the poor. He claims that one's own utility can be increased by giving to the poor if one cares about the welfare of those who are less fortunate. Traditional economic theory relies on markets to allocate resources efficiently and public policy to use taxes and subsidies to redistribute income to the poor. Rice contends, however, that there are no true taxes or subsidies that are politically acceptable, so the use of market competition is problematic because of the existence of the externality of consumption. If income is not redistributed, the market is inefficient, because people will still want the poor to have more than they already do; if income is redistributed, though, then traditional economics says that efficiency is compromised.[76]

How do the externalities relate to health care? Rice suggests that the large uninsured population causes a negative externality of consumption: A lack of insurance, or even inadequate insurance, can cause situations where people see themselves as less fortunate compared with others. The greater the disparity between those who have insurance and those who do not will lead to even more of the negative externalities.[77] This same scenario can also lead to positive externalities: People with insurance and concern for others may seek remedies to ensure that those without insurance are able to obtain coverage.[78] These remedies may take the form of some type of public policy to guarantee that those who need medical care can obtain it even if they do not have adequate financial means to pay for it—a policy that does not rely on market forces. Medicare and Medicaid are examples of this type of public policy.

In addition to causing negative externalities, Rice argues that market competition may not bring about the highest level of societal welfare because market theory erroneously relies on the assumption that consumer tastes are predetermined when they enter the marketplace.[79] He contends that in traditional market theory, consumer preferences are thought to be immutable and predetermined outside of the economic system in which a person lives. Rice challenges this assumption by arguing that people's decisions are influenced by their environments. He points to the use of advertising by the media to influence people's purchasing decisions.

Rice gives three examples of consumer behaviors that are not predetermined but are the result of environmental factors. In the case where a person is addicted to a substance, say cigarettes, this person's demand for cigarettes is much higher than that of someone who is not addicted to them.[80]

Rice's second example is "habit formed by past consumption patterns."[81] In the traditional market model, people are assumed to know what is best for them and then demand it. Rice contends that certain tastes, such as in music, are formed by prior experiences and the economic environment in which the individual has lived, and that someone's current tastes will also determine purchasing decisions in the future. It is difficult for people with set tastes and other ingrained behavior to care to know what alternatives exist, even ones that might make them better off.

Rice's third type of consumer behavior that is not predetermined is occupational choice. Rice suggests that people are often forced to work certain jobs because they are limited in alternatives. One may live in a small town where there is one factory that employs most of the town's population. One may take a cleaning job because it seems to be the only job available at the time. These choices do not reflect predetermination but a lack of alternatives.[82]

If consumer tastes are not predetermined, then advertising takes on great importance. Rice contends that there are two types of advertising: One provides objective information, such as the price of a product, and the other attempts to change consumer tastes. The information contained in advertisements is not necessarily in the best interest of consumers.

Furthermore, if tastes are not predetermined, then health care can be influenced through education, often through a government agency. Rice gives the example of smoking.[83] The federal government has taken several measures simply to reduce tobacco consumption. There has long been a ban on the advertising of tobacco products on television, and there is an antismoking campaign. Tobacco companies are required by law to place health disclaimers on packaging.

Rice sees cost control as an even larger issue if, indeed, consumer health wants and behaviors are malleable. Many experts claim the increased use of medical technology is a major contributor to rising medical costs. Because consumer tastes are the result of previous experiences, then people are more likely to demand new technologies because they constantly expect them. Certain high-tech procedures, such as coronary bypass and angioplasty, are so readily available in the United States that people have come to expect to use them. But these technologies may not necessarily reflect increasing utility levels, as traditional market theory would propose. Studies show that people in countries that spend far less on medical technologies are actually happier with their health care systems.[84]

Rice challenges a third assumption of traditional market theory: that a person is the best judge of his or her own welfare. He concludes that this is not necessarily the case, pointing to laws that limit an individual's choice in matters that may seem to pertain only to his or her own person, such as laws forbidding the selling of one's organs, the purchase of narcotics, and the solicitation of a prostitute.[85] Such limits indicate that society does not deem people always to be the best judges of their own welfare.

The fourth and fifth assumptions Rice calls into question concern consumer information. In traditional economic theory consumer information plays a key role. In order to maximize the utility of their purchases, consumers must have adequate information, and they must know the results of their consumption decisions. Rice examines several studies showing little evidence that consumers understand alternatives in the health care market. One study showed that consumers were particularly bad at understanding their health care plans.[86] Another major problem area for consumers is in using report cards to help them choose health plans. Report cards weigh several plan factors, such as quality, flexibility, and costs, but report cards vary considerably both in their comprehensibility as well as in their effectiveness.[87]

Related to this but occuring after care is received are *counterfactual questions*, through which a health care provider asks a patient what he or she thinks would have happened had history been different and had the patient made different choices in seeking diagnosis, receiving treatment, and so on. Rice contends that it is very difficult for the patient to answer this type of question, which is frequently asked by medical offices and clinics to determine whether consumers think they made the right decisions. For example, a person goes to a specialist for a dermatology condition. After receiving treatment, the patient is surveyed regarding what would have happened had he or she not sought the care of the particular specialist. What if the patient had seen a primary care doctor instead of the specialist? What might have happened had the patient seen a different specialist from the one actually seen? What if he or she had not seen a physician at all?[88] It is often difficult enough to judge the results of a health care decision, much less compare them with hypothetical outcomes.

Another assumption Rice questions is the notion that people are rational. He acknowledges that defining *rational* is a precarious undertaking, but he uses the theory of cognitive dissonance to make his point of what rational behavior is *not*. *Cognitive dissonance* exists when a person has inconsistent or contradictory knowledge, beliefs, or behaviors at more or less the same time. Many people smoke while knowing that it is harmful to their health, and Rice contends that such behavior could not be defined as "rational."[89] Certain economists have used cognitive dissonance in describing particular economic behaviors, such as the refusal to save enough money for retirement. People simply do not wish to think about their old age, and they simply refuse to cut back on their current spending to save for retirement. Rice suggests that this is one reason the government of the United States has established the Social Security and Medicare programs.[90]

Traditional economic theory also relies on the assumption that people reveal their preferences through their actions. Rice analyzes the work of economist Amartya Sen, who addresses the theory of revealed preference in several works. Sen argues that people can be motivated by feelings of sympathy or commitment to a cause, which can "drive a wedge between personal choice and personal welfare."[91] Thus, people can act for reasons other than "selfishness," and their choices may not result in any direct personal benefit. Rice contends that an individual may choose something that improves social but not his or her own personal welfare; on the other hand, a person may choose not to help others even when it would improve one's own welfare somehow.[92] Hence, an individual's actions may not reveal preferences (may not reveal, that is, self-oriented preferences because they are "obscured" by expressing preferences for the common good).

Such attitudes sometimes manifest themselves in the health care arena. An individual might give money to a health care charity even though it does not improve his or her own utility directly but because he or she feels it is better for society. Or a person may want to give to a health care charity but does not do so because he or she feels that the charity is not solvent. In both scenarios the individual's own utility is not reflected by his or her market behavior.

Next Rice challenges the assumption in traditional economic theory that social welfare is based solely on individual utility, which is in turn reflected solely by goods and services consumed. He says that this assumption is based on a philosophical argument and gives two reasons to question its validity. The first comes, again, from the work of Amartya Sen, and Rice explains Sen's argument as follows. The traditional model does not distinguish between various qualities of utility. For example, if an individual gets pleasure from another's unhappiness, that pleasure has the same weight as any other pleasure. Sen suggests that perhaps society should be more concerned about more lofty desires. Another problem Sen finds with the traditional model assumption is the definition of an individual's welfare. He contends that defining it merely by the goods that the individual possesses is far too narrow. Goods do not reflect other important aspects of life, such as freedom.[93]

The second reason Rice gives against the assumption that social welfare can be defined by goods and services consumed comes from economist Robert Frank.[94] Frank argues that individuals are driven by status. Yet, status is relative in nature, so one individual's status increases in comparison with another individual's, which declines. Frank claims that this causes a situation that does not add to social welfare at all. The purchaser of a nice car will get utility from both the car itself as well as having a nicer car than someone else. When other people buy the same car, then the second part of the original purchaser's utility is canceled out, so that total utility, or social welfare, is lower than the sum of individual utilities.

Another assumption from traditional market theory that Rice challenges: Firms maximize their profits. Rice argues that this assumption does not apply to the health care industry for two major reasons. First, many health care providers are nonprofit entities. This is particularly the case for hospitals: In 2001 only 10 percent of all hospitals in the United States were for profit.[95] Furthermore, people who manage health service industries may be interested in attaining certain quality management objectives rather than maximizing overall profits.[96]

The next assumption that Rice challenges is the existence of increasing returns to scale. Earlier in this chapter I discussed returns to scale. If there are increasing returns to scale, the average cost of production will decrease while the number of producers supplying part of the output declines, eventually ending up at one producer supplying all of the output. As noted earlier, the implication of constant or decreasing returns to scale is that there is no advantage to having a monopoly. Rice suggests, however, that in the hospital sector there may be increasing returns to scale. He refers to a study by Stephen Finkler that examined economies of scale for open-heart procedures. Finkler found evidence for increasing returns to scale, because the average costs of these procedures did not bottom out until a hospital had performed about 500 procedures per year. Finkler concluded that costs could be saved by regionalizing open-heart surgery so that only a few facilities would provide the service.[97] Rice also points out that most medical experts agree that the patients of hospitals and physicians who perform a higher volume of a particular procedure have better health outcomes after the procedure, the mortality rates being lower.[98] If the average costs of certain specialty procedures are lower only after a higher volume and the health outcomes are better with a higher volume, that is an indication that increasing returns to scale are found in at least some areas of the health care industry.

Rice disputes traditional economic theory's assumption that there is no relationship between production and wealth distribution. If people do not have adequate food, he argues, then they are not likely to be very productive in the workforce. Also, people who are poor tend to be less healthy, which also affects their productivity at work.[99]

The final assumption that Rice addresses is the notion that the distribution of wealth is approved of by society. This concept is rooted in utilitarian philosophy, which does not evaluate economic systems on the basis of equity or fairness but on the theory that the possession of goods gives people utility, which gives society utility. Society is, therefore, viewed as merely an aggregate of all individuals. Rice provides a long critique of this assumption, finding three major faults with it. First, the assumption is too narrow and fails to recognize any issues related to social justice. Second, the assumption holds that people are driven solely by ownership of goods. Such a viewpoint is atomistic and ignores other aspects of the person. Finally, the assumption purports that the optimal redistribution of wealth should be in the form of cash grants instead of a transfer of goods or services themselves. Rice argues that in the health care sector it is better to redistribute wealth through goods and services. Among several reasons: People may not spend cash in a way that is best for them, and cash incentives may actually diminish work productivity by acting as incentives not to work.[100]

In his conclusion Thomas Rice states, "Why is there no reason to believe that a competitive marketplace will result in the best outcomes [for health care]? Because such a conclusion is based on many strong assumptions being met. This book examined over a dozen of the assumptions that need to be fulfilled to ensure that a free market results in the best outcomes for society; none of them were even close to being met in the health services."[101] Rice suggests that competition be viewed as just one possible policy alternative instead of being presumed to be the best policy. He supports a greater reliance on supply-side controls instead of demand-side controls, which are prevalent in free markets.

But what do other economists have to say about all of this?

The Yea-Sayers

The next chapter will look at the proposed health plans of four economists who are market advocates. Each of these plans reflects reasons why the market is precisely the best entity to oversee the provision of health care. First, however, let's look at one particularly well-written essay that defends the use of the market in the provision of health care. In "What Does Economics Have to Say about Health Policy Anyway? A Comment and Correction on Evans and Rice," economists Martin Gaynor and William Vogt specifically respond to some of the critiques Canadian economists Robert Evans and Thomas Rice make about the use of the market in the provision of health care. Here I will focus on their response to Rice and his arguments, which I laid out in the previous section.

Gaynor and Vogt begin their essay by stating, "The fact that health care markets are not textbook competitive markets is not news to economists."[102] The first challenge they make to Rice's critique is to clarify that the Pareto principle will not always differentiate between two alternatives. To explain this point, they use the example of two people who each prefer one product over the other. Sally prefers A to B, and Bob prefers B to A. In such a case the Pareto principle does not indicate which alternative is better.[103] Gaynor and Vogt also contend that there are often several Pareto optimal choices, each with a different distribution of wealth.[104] Third, they claim that the Pareto principle only suggests which alternative is better from the point of view of the members of a society. Hence, if a policy planner thinks that the consumption of certain products is good for society but if the members of that society agree that they do not want to consume those products, then the Pareto principle will call for a lower consumption level of the products that the people choose not to consume.[105] Finally, Gaynor and Vogt contend that the idea of a preference, as used in the Pareto principle, depends solely on how people would act, not on any external measure of what might be good for them.[106]

Next Gaynor and Vogt challenge Rice's argument that the Pareto principle should not be used for evaluation purposes. They argue that economics is no more or less normative than other fields, such as engineering.[107] Gaynor and Vogt challenge Rice's assertion that the Pareto principle cannot take into account people's status in society. They claim that when status is important, the change in total utility includes both a gain for the person buying the status product as well as a loss to another's utility for the envy he or she feels. A change in total utility is calculated by adding up all of the effects of a particular consumer action on everyone's utilities. Gaynor and Vogt point out that there are economic models showing that relative rankings are important and in which the Pareto optimum may be calculated.[108]

Gaynor and Vogt then address Rice's claims that Pareto criteria do not apply when people have preferences determined by their past experiences and that perfect competition does not work well under these circumstances. They argue that this is not the case, noting that "these sorts of dynamic effects in preferences are consistent with the standard textbook competitive models of economic behavior, so that Pareto optima are well defined and have their usual interpretation."[109] Moreover, with regard to addictive behaviors and their relationship to preference theory, in the mind of these economists, such preferences count the same as any other. Gaynor and Vogt criticize Rice for claiming "that the addict might be 'better-off' if she is forced to stop. . . . No support is provided for this judgment, and it is far from obvious to us that the addict's pain of withdrawal is somehow less valid than any other motive for preference formation."[110]

The final Rice perspective on the Pareto principle that Gaynor and Vogt challenge is his claim that a policymaker may care about values other than goods and services, such as freedom, instead of Pareto rankings. They contend that in traditional economic theory all economists agree that Pareto rankings are not the only criteria for social choice, anyway.[111] Instead, the rankings are merely one important tool. They conclude that Pareto optimality "may not be the exclusive criterion one might use in assessing forms of economic organization, but it is likely to be a relevant criterion both to a hypothetical benevolent social planner and to any real social planner."[112] Knowledge of the Pareto rankings is useful to any policy planner since resources must be allocated to finance the goal of the planner.

The next issue that Gaynor and Vogt address is Rice's argument that it is better to distribute wealth through in-kind transfers rather than cash transfers. They argue that with in-kind transfer the poor must either use the health services or nothing. With the alternative, cash transfers allow the poor to show their preference by either buying health services or spending the money on something else.

To illustrate the costs of such a policy choice, Gaynor and Vogt take the example of coronary artery bypass graft surgery.[113] This surgery costs about $25,000, and they say that in many instances the procedure is done solely to alleviate the pain of angina. The Pareto criterion requires that the poor person be paid the $25,000, which he or she can spend either to pay for the surgery or for some other purpose. Rice would require that the poor person receive the surgery as an in-kind transfer plan, but suppose the poor person would rather live with the pain of angina and have the option of using the money for something else. Under these circumstances, Rice's plan would make the person worse off, according to the poor individual him- or herself, than would the cash transfer. Gaynor and Vogt point out that the Pareto criterion does not necessarily make the right choice for an individual, but deviations from it always result in frustrating someone's preferences, which could be satisfied at no cost to anyone else. They also contend that it is usually the poor who suffer from this inefficiency, since they are often the target of such policies and are rarely in a position to avoid them.

Gaynor and Vogt address Rice's claim that assessing preferences is very problematic because of insufficient consumer information and the possibility of some indirect effects. They suggest that "people make decisions under uncertainty all of the time, and by necessity some will turn out badly ex post."[114] Regarding the possibility of indirect effects and externalities of consumption, Gaynor and Vogt acknowledge that there are limitations of standard demand theory and that these limitations are recognized by economists. Still, they argue, the existence of these limitations does not render a "blanket condemnation" of demand theory.[115] Rather, the circumstances under which these limitations occur are being studied by economists and should continue being studied. As an example of such ongoing research, Gaynor and Vogt mention the progress that has been made in drawing inferences about the structure of costs, demand, and competition solely from data on prices and quantities.[116]

Gaynor and Vogt conclude their essay by stating that although they defend the use of Pareto optimality and demand theory in health care economics, they acknowledge that these tools are not perfect. They suggest, though, that these tools are still the best available to date for assessing people's preferences. Moreover, they claim there will never be a perfect tool, so economists must use the tools they have, with the understanding that they have certain flaws.

Market Mechanisms

Many politicians, as well as the popular media, simplify the debate over who should fund and organize health care. They often reduce the arguments to a "government versus the market" theme. In practice the issues are much more complicated. Health care systems are so vast, and they involve such complex management and decision-making problems at so many levels, that the application of market mechanisms to health care is filled with conceptual as well as practical problems.

A number of practices are frequently used in health care, though, including patient choice, negotiated contracts, and open bidding for contracts. Market practices can be used to control price of services or market share. They can be adopted to influence different sectors within health care systems, such as the funding of health care, the production of health care, and the distribution of funds to service providers. Market incentives can be used to influence the behavior of physicians, nurses, and support staff.

The precise role that market mechanisms should play in a socially responsible health care system remains hotly debated. Hence, there are many varying models of health care throughout the world. Some systems are hybrid, representing a combination of market mechanisms with government ownership. Others have a strong government presence and use only a few market mechanisms, such as user fees, to help fund the system. Others, like in the United States, rely heavily on market mechanisms and competition. The most commonly used market mechanisms are private insurance, managed care, user fees, physician incentives, and health accounts.

Private Insurance

Private insurance is generally used to finance health care through premiums paid by the individual who is the insured, by the employer of the insured, or shared between the insured and the employer. The cost of the premium is determined in one of three ways. It may be individually rated, based on an assessment of the chances that the individual may require health care. It may be community rated, determined by an estimate of the health risks of a geographically defined population. It may be group rated, based on estimates considering the risks associated with all of the employees in a single organization.

Private insurance has several potential advantages over other market mechanisms.[117] It enables wealthier people to buy policies to pay for their own health care. This, in turn, allows government to use public resources to provide health care for the poor and others who do not have access to private insurance. Private insurance, because of its competitive nature, is thought to encourage efficiency, creativity, and individual responsibility. It is also thought to offer people more choices and personal input regarding their health care.

On the other hand, private insurance has many disadvantages, particularly if it is unregulated.[118] An unregulated health insurance market does not work well for many reasons. People in poor health have preexisting conditions that may make it difficult or even impossible to obtain private insurance. If people withhold information about their health from the insurance company, this would skew the insurance risk pool. In a related matter, insurance companies often lack complete information about the current health of a person who is already insured and cannot know all necessary information about activities that may affect his or her future health. For example, once an individual has insurance he or she may start participating in risky, health-threatening behavior. How can the insurance company know this? Estimating a future claim and calculating risks become very problematic, which, in turn, makes rating a premium difficult.

Even if private insurance is regulated, as it is in the United States, it is still problematic. Private insurance, with its ability to rate risks by age group, tends to discriminate in favor of younger, healthier adults, who do not use the health care system a lot. For the same reason, premiums for the elderly, who often need insurance coverage the most, are quite high and may be unaffordable. It is also highly desirable for insurance companies to spread their financial risk across large numbers of people. This encourages insurers to market their plans only to groups, but, for various reasons, many people do not qualify for group plans, and the cost of individual plans is out of their reach. Community rating of health insurance is often seen as a tool to guarantee fairness. Yet, when the purchase of insurance is voluntary, people who are healthy, and therefore good insurance risks, may consider the community-rated premium too expensive and leave the pool to self-insure. By leaving, they drive up the cost of the community-rated premium, which in turn gradually makes the insurance less affordable to those who are in poorer health or less affluent.[119]

For the reader to appreciate the various ways private insurance works, the following sections briefly describe different health care systems in certain nations.

United States. Before the enactment of Medicare and Medicaid in the mid-1960s, Americans who could not afford medical care generally relied on charity. With the occurrence of the major changes in medicine in the first part of the twentieth century, which were discussed earlier in this chapter, paying for medical care became an issue for middle-class Americans. As a response to this situation, private insurance was developed. Several different kinds of health plans were adapted, from voluntary "sick funds" organized by organizations to help immigrants, fraternal clubs, and unions. Blue Cross was created for individuals to pool their risks of incurring major hospital expenses by paying small monthly payments that would then cover hospitalization costs.[120]

Private health insurance grew rapidly in the twentieth century because of benefits offered in the workplace and favorable tax treatments of employers' contributions to health benefit plans.[121] By 1940 half of the states had adopted legal frameworks for hospital service-benefit plans, which established state insurance commissioners to review insurance plan rates, and insurance plans were exempted from taxes as charitable organizations.[122] In that same year, Blue Cross had an enrollment of more than 6 million people, and another 3.7 million people were covered by commercial insurers.[123] By 1953, 29 percent of all Americans were covered by for-profit commercial carriers, 27 percent by the nonprofit Blue Cross, and 7 percent by independent plans.[124] Toward the end of that decade, almost two-thirds of the population in the United States had some type of insurance coverage.[125]

Enrollment in insurance plans began to slow in the 1960s.[126] Then the enactment of the Medicare and Medicaid programs expanded insurance coverage and filled much of the gap in insurance coverage. However, with rising costs of medical care in the 1970s and 1980s, cost controls were instigated at all levels of the provision of medical care. Cost controls met with some success in the 1990s, but the number of individuals with private insurance declined and has continued to decline. In 2004 there were 44.5 million Americans without any type of health insurance.

Private insurance has been key to providing access to health care for many Americans as well as revenue for health care providers. In 2001 approximately $375.1 billion was spent by private insurers on health care, representing per capita spending of $2,484.[127] Overall, health care spending in the United States was $4,370 per person, representing a hefty 15 percent of the GDP. In 2003 job-based insurance covered almost 175 million people and their dependents who were actively working, 3 million early retirees, and 12 million people who were eligible for Medicare.[128]

Still, the cost of insurance to the employee is increasing annually. Between 2000 and 2003, nominal employee contribution for coverage had risen 50 percent for single coverage and 49 percent for family coverage.[129] With the increasing cost of private insurance, it is difficult to imagine that the number of uninsured will decrease anytime soon.

Switzerland. Before 1996 private health insurance in Switzerland was voluntary and individual. Premiums were relatively low because they were supported by general tax subsidies. The proportion of subsidies in relation to expenditures had declined in the mid-1970s, which resulted in higher premiums. Health care costs also rose in the 1980s, which caused premiums to increase even further.

In 1996 the Health Insurance Act established a system of compulsory health insurance for all residents of Switzerland. Under this act, insurance is provided by nonprofit insurance funds. The funds are not government-controlled social insurance funds, but they are regulated by government. Every fund must accept all who apply for coverage and charge the same premiums to all insurees (although different insurers can charge different amounts). Furthermore, a mandatory basic coverage must be offered by all insurers. In certain cantons (or states) where premiums exceed 8 to 10 percent of a person's income, the federal government helps subsidize the excess cost.[130] Private insurance policies may be purchased for additional coverage.

This program has provided Swiss residents with universal coverage but has had cost control problems. In 2001 Switzerland spent the equivalent of $3,222 U.S. dollars per person on health care.[131] This reflects 10.9 percent of the nation's GDP, one of the highest rates in Europe.

Australia. Historically, Australia's health care system has alternated between public and private insurance and between free and fee-based health care.[132] Since 1975 all Australian citizens and permanent residents are covered by a national health insurance program that provides comprehensive coverage. It is funded by both the federal government and the six state governments. Private insurance is purchased as an additional option to the national plan.

People choose to purchase private insurance so they can choose their physicians in particular hospitals and upgrade their hospital accommodations. In 1998 approximately 30 percent of Australians were enrolled in private insurance plans.[133] The federal government oversees the insurance industry by regulating the costs of premiums and the types of benefits that are offered. Insurers are required to have certain minimum financial reserves and are required to pay for a consumer complaint bureau. There are also controls on contracting between private insurers and hospitals.[134] The purchase of private health insurance decreased in the 1990s, which resulted in the federal government's introducing policies to encourage its use. One such policy provided that individuals get a 30 percent rebate for premiums paid for private health insurance. Other policies provided for selective contracting and a move away from community rating in premium determination.[135]

The early statistics on the impact of the policies suggest that private insurance enrollment is increasing.[136] Yet, it remains to be seen whether a substantial shift of resources from the public sector to the private sector will occur or whether there will be declining support for the universal health insurance that the nation currently has. Some experts contend that government's promotion of private insurance is more consistent with a philosophy that private insurance is a competitor of universal health insurance rather than a supplement to it.[137]

Summary of Private Insurance. It is difficult to characterize the role that private insurance plays in health care around the world, because every country's system is unique. For countries that have government-mandated universal health care programs, there are two major issuesconcerning private insurance. First, what, exactly, is the role of private insurers? Second, should private insurers be able to compete against each other?[138] For some countries there are issues of fairness and efficiency. Private health insurance can be a contributing factor in making the financing of health care a regressive system.

Generally, access to private health care is determined either by an individual's ability to pay or, if the individual is employed, by the employer's desire and ability to pay. Thus, a gap may exist in coverage. For example, in the United States, the very poor and elderly may qualify for federal Medicare or Medicaid. People working at higher-paying jobs, especially, may receive insurance benefits through their work. The wealthy can also purchase their own private insurance. Yet, it is the "working poor" who are most often without any type of health care coverage, because they cannot get coverage through their employment or afford to purchase individual policies. It is estimated that 80 percent of the uninsured in America are from families whose head of household works full- or part-time.[139]

There is some evidence to support the argument that private insurance is a very efficient system. Government-run health care programs are restricted by more supply-side controls, such as fixed budgets, budget caps, and restrictive use of expensive technologies. These controls can result in waiting lists where patients must wait up to several weeks for a procedure that would be done in a matter of days in the United States, with its system of private insurance. Canada has gained notoriety for its waiting lists. A *New Times* survey conducted in 2003 found major increases in waiting times: Orthopedic surgery had a median waiting time of 32 weeks; ophthalmology, 27 weeks; neurosurgery, 17 weeks; and gynecology, 17 weeks.[140] Still, a survey showed that 90 percent of Canadians questioned were satisfied with the system.[141]

Managed Care

Managed care has existed in the United States for over seventy years. As early as 1932, the Committee on the Costs of Medical Care argued that medical practices should be organized into prepaid group practices.[142] This type of system, whose group practices came to be called health maintenance organizations, or HMOs, would serve as an alternative to the "fee for service" system, which dominated health care in the United States until the 1970s.

Today there is a variety of managed care systems. One system is based on the preferred provider organization (PPO), is a group of physicians who form an organization in order to contract with a variety of insurers to provide care for their insurees, generally at a reduced fee. The insured can usually choose his or her primary care physician from among those in the PPO and pay them a copayment for their services. A patients may also go to physicians who are not within the PPO, but the amount of coverage will be reduced.[143]

The best-known managed care system, though, is the HMO, whose insurance plan differs from traditional indemnity insurance plans. Rather than paying for doctor's fees, hospitals, and pharmacies after it has provided its services, an HMO actually provides most of the medical care for its enrollees. In other words, an HMO acts as both the provider of health insurance and the deliverer of medical services. Theoretically, this type of system allows for more control over costs and delivery of services.

As mentioned earlier, with the rising health care costs in the late 1960s and early 1970s, President Nixon initiated legislation that encouraged the development of HMOs. The HMO Act of 1973 was signed into law to encourage the use of HMOs. It provided $375 million for HMO development, subsidized HMO premiums, and required private employers with 25 or more employees to offer HMO plans.[144] The act's original intent was to control health care costs by efficient management and to provide integrated care. HMOs may be for-profit or nonprofit organizations. For decades they were predominantly nonprofit. By 2002, however, 62.7 percent of HMOs were for-profit organizations.[145]

There are many variations of HMOs, but they can be sorted into two model categories.[146] The staff model is set up so that the health entity pays the physician's salary; provides the necessary support staff and support systems, such as equipment and office space; and provides prescription drugs. This model provides hospitalization either in the HMO's own hospital or through arrangements with other hospitals. With the other model, the independent practice association model, the HMO contracts with associations or groups of physicians to care for the patients that the HMO insures. The contracted physicians then provide their own offices, support staff, and support systems. The HMO usually pays the physicians a fixed amount to treat the patients covered by the contract, and then the association pays its physicians for taking care of the covered patients. However, there are variances in the way the physicians are paid. Often certain mechanisms known as physician incentives are used to encourage physicians to control costs. These will be discussed later.

HMOs have been very successful in some ways and a dismal failure in others. Several studies in the mid-nineties showed that for a while HMOs were able to control health care costs. On the average, rate premiums were lower, and lengths of hospital stays were shorter. The prevalence of HMOs was also credited with limiting the use of high-tech medical equipment in the nineties. The number of magnetic resonance imaging (MRI) units across the United States was reduced, thereby lowering costs and emphasizing the development of lower-cost technologies.[147]

The ability of HMOs to control costs and provide efficient services became even stronger with intense competition between them. Large concentrations of HMOs in particular regions around the United States increased the competition for enrollees. Large employers shopped around for the best HMO deals. There was competition in factors besides price, as well. The size of the HMO network, the style of care, and even the quality of care all became competitive factors. HMOs have come to dominate the health care landscape. As of 2003, 95 percent of people with employer-sponsored health care were enrolled in some type of managed health care plan.[148]

But HMOs have not been able to maintain their positive momentum. There has been a tremendous amount of criticism of HMOs on several fronts. Patient as well as physician complaints about access to specialists, choice of health plans, and quality of care have become commonplace. This has led to legislation requiring HMOs to provide denied or restricted services and force them to stop the use of "gag clauses." There have also been a multitude of legal actions over HMOs' accountability to patients.

Because the HMO Act of 1973 was a federal law, however, the Employee Retirement Income Security Act of 1974 (ERISA) governs such lawsuits, so patients are forbidden to file lawsuits against HMOs in state courts. Much to the dismay of many HMO enrollees, ERISA limits the amount of damages in a lack-of-care claim, thereby significantly reducing the amount of compensation that a patient might otherwise receive. In 2004 the U.S. Supreme Court upheld the requirement that HMO patients must file claims in federal court under ERISA and cannot sue in state courts.[149]

The backlash against HMOs has also led to a movement to get Congress to enact a patients' rights bill that would regulate HMOs' behavior. In 2001 the Senate passed its own version of legislation that the House had passed earlier, giving patients broad authority to sue HMOs, allowing patients direct access to specialists, and requiring HMOs to cover visits to the nearest emergency room. In fall 2003, negotiations between the House and the Senate on the patients' rights bill were deemed at an impasse, and the legislation was considered dead.[150] Similar legislation was introduced in May 2005; both the House and the Senate bills remained in committee throughout the remainder of the congressional term.

There is a lot of speculation about what happened to the cost-cutting effectiveness of HMOs. Frankly, what HMOs did to control costs was to ration health care. Although it appeared initially that they were quite successful at keeping costs down, several studies showed that the major reason HMOs were able to do this was because they produced significantly lower hospital admission rates, compared to indemnity plans.[151] In fact, HMOs gained notoriety for their policies that simply restrict a patient's access to health care by limiting the diagnostic tests that a physician can order; limiting medications that a physician can prescribe; limiting the ability of a patient to see specialists; limiting second opinions; and limiting the number of days a patient can be hospitalized, as well as limiting the choice of hospitals.[152]

Moreover, between 1996 and 2003, the average annual premium rates for HMOs rose about as fast as the rates for all types of plans, 8 percent per year.[153] The copayment amount that workers pay also increased.[154] Statistics such as these caused health care economist Alain Enthoven to declare that HMOs "did not bring about a fundamental reform in the way health care is organized and delivered. Managed care has broken down under an onslaught from lawyers, politicians, consumers, and doctors."[155]

In sum, it is difficult to say whether HMOs might have been able to control costs had external factors and heavy criticism not intervened. Still, two conclusions can be made. People in the United States do not want their ability to make health care choices restricted. Also, physicians in the United States do not want their clinical judgment restricted. The HMO experiment has brought an important policy question to the forefront: Can we have affordable health care and maintain the choices patients want and the freedom physicians want?

User Fees, Copayments, and Deductibles

User fees, also known as copayments, are one of the most prevalent forms of cost sharing in health care systems. User fees are even used in countries that have universal health care coverage. They encompass a large variety of charges, but the common characteristic they all share is the requirement that the patient pay for some part of what would otherwise be free care.[156] In the United States the term *copayment* is commonly used, and in other countries the term *user fee* is widely accepted. Hence, I will use the term *copayment* when specifically discussing the United States and *user fee* otherwise.

According to one economic theory, the basic reason for employing user fees is to decrease the demand for health services. Some economic theorists contend that the demand for health care exceeds socially desirable levels when services are completely covered by public or private insurance. User fees are therefore thought to force patients to consider costs before demanding health services.[157] On the other hand, some health policy analysts argue that it is inconsistent public policy to use a method that increases revenue as a way to control costs.[158] They claim that if the health care provider induces demand, and patient spending is equal to provider revenue, then cost sharing will not decrease costs. Rather, it will cause the costs to be shifted to those who are sick and need medical care and therefore use the health care system more.

In the United States, demand-side cost controls are becoming more and more common. This is evidenced by an increasing amount of health care costs being paid for by employees. One common method of cost shifting is the use of copayments, which the vast majority of employees with work-related health care plans pay. Moreover, employees with a $20 copayment for a visits to the physician's office rose 19 percent in 2003 and 27 percent in 2004. Copayments for pharmaceuticals have also risen sharply; in recent years many employers have increased the cost of prescription drug copayments significantly, from $5 to $10 for generic drugs and $15 to $50 for nongeneric drugs.[159]

Another striking example of employer-to-employee cost shifting is the increase in the amount of annual deductibles that are paid by employees. A deductible is paid by the insurance enrollee before the insurance policy will begin paying for a covered medical expense. Average annual deductibles have skyrocketed over the past several years. Between 1988 and 2004, the average annual deductible for covered workers under a conventional family insurance plan went from $375 to $861 per year.[160] Within networks that do not have specified contracted providers, the average deductible for a family went from $177 in 1988 to $558 in 2004.[161]

There seems to be no end in sight for increases in employee cost sharing. In a recent survey done by the Kaiser Family Foundation, employers were asked whether they plan to make changes in their employees' health care plans in the near future. Fully 52 percent of all large firms (those with 200 or more workers) and 15 percent of all small firms (those with 3 to 199 workers) answered that they are "very likely" to increase employee contributions by next year.[162]

Most countries in Europe use cost sharing to raise revenue or control health care costs for physicians and hospital services. It is also used for prescription drugs but generally not for the young or old.[163] European countries seem very concerned about protecting the income of its citizens, though. Almost all European countries limit the amount of out-of-pocket expenses that an individual or family will have to pay for health care costs. Also, unlike with most health care plans in the United States, in Europe it is extremely rare to find health care benefit maximums or restrictions on the amount a health care service can be utilized.[164] In Belgium a person considered low-income is eligible to receive an exemption from health care cost sharing. In Austria low-income people do not have to pay user fees for pharmaceuticals. In France people who have any one of 30 diseases considered serious or chronic are exempt from user fees.[165]

In developing countries, user fees are not uncommon. In Ethiopia, Namibia, and South Africa, national user fees have existed for many years. Since 1980 many other African countries have adopted user fees due to World Bank requirements.[166] The following are the objectives of implementing user fees in these countries: to raise revenue, to improve quality of health care, to extend covered services, to promote efficient health care, and to improve equity of health care.[167] Although the impact of user fee requirements is not yet determined, some generalizations can be made. The imposition of user fees appears to reduce the utilization of health care. This is especially true for the poor. For example, in Zimbabwe, UNICEF reported, twice as many women were dying in childbirth in the capital city's Harare Hospital in 1993 than those who died prior to the implementation of user fees in 1990. UNICEF also found that fewer people were visiting clinics and hospitals. It concluded that one reason for the decrease in visits was that patients could not afford to pay the user fees.[168]

Also, user fees in developing countries may actually encourage inefficiency. This is particularly the case when the revenue from fees is kept at the same place that it is collected. In addition, there is a pattern of lack of coordination within the fee system itself. Sometimes lower levels within a health care system charge higher fees than higher levels. This practice encourages a greater use of services that are less cost effective.[169]

Finally, user fees in developing countries raise questions of equity. Systems that rely entirely on user fees rather than any type of risk sharing or prepayment are likely to restrict access to health care. Moreover, user fees do not generate enough revenue to assist with improving health care for the poor. They may, however, help pay for costs, except for salaries, in lower-level health facilities.[170]

Attempts to use sliding-scale user fees to make health care more accessible to the poor also appear to be ineffective. Many experts suggest that they in fact benefit the more wealthy members of developing countries.[171]

To summarize: Most economists agree that user fees limit access to health care for the poor unless they are accompanied by exemptions or other forms of compensatory assistance, because fees use up a larger proportion of the household incomes of the poor than those of people of greater means. Moreover, the elderly, the young, and the chronically ill are negatively affected by user fees. For these groups of people utilization costs are more of a deterrent than for healthy people, simply because they need to use the health care system more.[172] Finally, user fees cause inequity in the financing of health care, because the burden of costs falls primarily on the poor and the unhealthy.

Physician Incentives

Another form of market mechanism in health care is physician compensation. The numerous methods of compensation can be reduced to three categories: fee for service, salary, and capitation. Fee for service, for years the method of choice, is a simple concept. The physician or other health care provider performs services for the patient, then bills either the patient or the patient's insurance company, and the fee is paid.

However, there are three major problems with this system. Neither the patient nor the third-party payer has any control over the amount of the fee. The physician or other health care provider has sole control over the type and amount of service rendered, along with the cost. Also, a fee-for-service system has no built-in cost controls. To the contrary, there is a high incentive for health care providers to raise their fees to make more money. Traditionally, when government, through Medicare and Medicaid, and private insurance companies are paying the fees, they pay whatever is "customary," which is determined by what others in the profession charge. Hence, whenever some physicians or hospitals increase their fees, the others follow, thereby making the new, higher fee the customary fee. When private individuals are paying for their own health care, providers are fairly sensitive to what they can afford. When an "anonymous" third-party institutions are paying, the fees rapidly increase.[173] Lastly, because there are no incentives to limit the use of health care resources, a fee-for-service system is believed to encourage the overuse of health care.

Therefore, the fee-for-service system has been almost entirely replaced by one of two other mechanisms. The second type of physician compensation is a salary, whereby a physician is paid a given amount per month or per year regardless of how many patients he or she treats. Salaries are commonly found in HMOs. Capitation, another common method of compensation, is often used in managed care. A prepayment for the potential use of services is made, whether or not any service is rendered. Generally, the physician receives a fixed fee per member enrolled in the health plan, and the physician must try to provide a set of services that, on average, stays within the fixed amount. For example, a physician may agree to provide medical treatment for 750 people for one year for $75,000. The physician will get paid that amount regardless of how much care the 750 people actually need or receive during that year.[174]

Three physician incentive variations are the use of bonuses, subcapitation, and fee withhold. These incentives are basically tools to stop physicians from overusing diagnostic tests, referrals, and other ancillary services.[175] Monetary bonuses are given when a physician meets certain criteria, such as a positive peer evaluation or a decrease in the cost of patient care. A health care provider who gets capitation monies for a group of patients may use subcapitation, subcontracting with other providers to provide services on a capitated basis. Fee withholds are delayed payments that are based on the physician's performance.[176] The use of these incentives has grown tremendously, with estimates that about half of all American physicians use some type of capitation or withhold plan.[177]

Physician incentives are controversial, but every system has some sort of financial incentive. Fee-for-service systems might encourage doctors to give more care than patients need. Salaried physicians may not work as hard as other doctors. Most of the incentive controversy, though, surrounds capitation, bonuses, and withholds. With capitation, physicians have an incentive to increase their number of patients while limiting medical services. Federal and state regulations have been adopted to try to prevent the most serious problems associated with capitation. For example, managed care organizations that contract with Medicare or Medicaid cannot place a physician at substantial financial risk with regard to incentives. "Stop-loss" protection must be provided when financial incentives place more than 25 percent of a physician's income at risk.[178]

Even though it is under fire, the physician incentive system remains very strong. But is it effective? In their book Callahan and Wasunna examine the effectiveness of physician incentives. They argue that three major questions should be explored in order to assess the effectiveness of incentives. First, do incentives actually increase physician productivity? Callahan and Wasunna cite a 2002 study that confirms an important finding of similar studies: Incentives do indeed increase productivity.[179]

Next, do incentives really contain costs? Much of the evidence to date shows that incentives do not contain costs. Rather, costs are directly related to the characteristics of the individuals enrolled in the plans and to the level of plan benefits. Costs actually increased with the age of the enrollee, with female enrollees, and along with the benefit amount of the health plan.[180]

A third issue regarding incentives is whether physicians' economic interest influences the care they provide patients. The most troublesome potential problem with incentives is that they might actually harm a patient by limiting his or her access to care. For example, in order to increase his or her incentive pay, a physician might deny important diagnostic tests. A physician may refuse to refer a patient to a specialist whose expertise is critical to the patient's care. Callahan and Wasunna concluded that "if such abuses occur, it is difficult in theory to prove and has not been proven in the few studies that exist. Even so, it remains a concern."[181] Indeed, this is a major concern in the health care community. There seems to be some agreement there that incentive arrangements should not put physicians' money at too high a risk and should therefore be implemented only within larger practices.

Another incentives issue, which does not get the attention its importance merits, is the effect of incentives on public perception of and confidence in the health care system. Even if incentives never actually affect a patient's care, there is a perception that they might. Such perceptions harm a patient's confidence in his or her physician, as well as in the health care system overall. The patient-doctor relationship is a very important one. It must be based on trust. Any erosion of that trust cannot have a positive effect on health care.[182]

The jury is still out on the effectiveness and impact, be it positive or negative, of the various physician incentives. Public perceptions remain skeptical. There have been several lawsuits over their use, and restrictive state and federal legislation has been enacted.[183] Regardless of what effect incentives actually have on the health care system, they do appear to erode public trust. Since trust in the health care system is an essential characteristic of a good system, physician incentives should be used very selectively and carefully.

Health Accounts

There are three types of health accounts. A health savings account (HSA) is a special account akin to an individual retirement account. It allows an individual with a high-deductible health plan to set up a tax-free account to pay for medical bills. A person under the age of sixty-five can set up an HSA to place up to $5,150 per year in a tax-free account to be used for medical expenses; an HSA has a minimum $2,000 deductible for a family. An HSA can be purchased through the individual's own health plan or through an independent health provider. The money does not have to be spent within the calendar year in which it was placed in the account, so any unused portion carries forward into the next year.

There were two precursors to HSAs. First, medical savings accounts (MSAs) were established by Congress in 1996. An individual could buy a high-deductible insurance plan and open up a special financial account, the MSA, to help to pay for the deductible or other medical costs. MSAs were not widely used, and by 2002 only 85,000 people had enrolled in such plans.[184] Hence, MSAs were terminated in January 2004 and replaced with HSAs in the 2003 Medicare Reform Bill.

The other predecessor to HSAs is the flexible spending account (FSA). An FSA, or flex account, allows an employee to put aside some of the pretax money from salaries or wages to pay for medical expenses. Flex accounts are quite common, with about seven million people using them.[185] They pose two major problems for individuals and their families, though. An FSA has a "use it or lose it" feature. The money placed in the account must be spent by the end of the same calendar year; it cannot be carried over into future years. Also, employers can determine the amount of money placed into an FSA and therefore can limit the amount to a rather low sum.

Although HSAs have been highly touted, employers have been particularly slow to offer them to their employees. One reason is that it took the Treasury Department months to sort through all of the issues that employers had about administering HSAs.[186] Moreover, large employers are concerned about how people with chronic conditions, such as diabetes, will fare with HSAs. Such employees might drain their savings accounts year after year, because they will continually pass the deductible.[187]

Other critics of HSAs charge that high-deductible insurance policies will cause people—especially those with low incomes, who have less disposable income—to delay needed medical care, because they will want to keep their money as long as possible. Moreover, critics also argue, HSAs are designed to encourage the active involvement of individuals in their medical decisions, but the average individual is not well equipped to decide what medical care is essential and what is not. In many instances, there is not sufficient information for people to make good health care decisions that are also cost-containing decisions.[188] Critics also contend that HSAs are relatively ineffective in controlling health care costs, because about 10 percent of people, often with chronic or multiple health problems, make up about 69 percent of overall health costs. These people will continue to have high health costs regardless of what incentives are presented to them to curb health care spending.[189] Finally, neither FSAs nor HSAs offer any incentives directed at controlling the supply side of health care.

Internationally, MSAs have been used in several countries with mixed success. Like the United States, South Africa has established private-sector MSAs. However, only about 20% of the population there has purchased private insurance, with about half of these plans consisting of MSAs.[190] Public MSAs can be found in China and Singapore. Although there is not much data on the success of the Chinese program, Singapore's MSAs have received a lot of attention. Singapore has a mandatory and universal MSA system that has been run by the federal government since 1984. The system has remained controversial and has had mixed results. Singapore spends a smaller amount on health care than many other nations (between 3 percent and 4 percent of the GDP), and many argue that the overall health of Singapore's citizens is quite good.[191] Yet, many attribute the relative success of MSAs in Singapore to its young population; strict supply controls on the use of technology, on prices of health services, and restricting the numbers of hospital beds, doctors, and specialists; and the population's high level of use of traditional medicine (folk and other alternative remedies), which is not paid for by government.[192]

The world of MSAs, HSAs, and FSAs is a mire of market mechanisms. Although each mechanism is intended to improve the health care system, the results are mixed. It appears that they do not have much impact on most health care systems. They can be used only by individuals who have fairly large disposable incomes. Moreover, they do not address health care demands that drive medical use and costs. Callahan and Wasunna sum them up when they write that they appear to be "more a symbol of market ambition than a useful device for holding down costs, improving efficiency, or enhancing equitable access."[193]

Various Countries' Responses to Market Mechanisms and Health Outcomes

In *Costs, Choice, and Equity: Medicine and the Market,* Callahan and Wasunna classify several countries according to their overall acceptance or rejection of market mechanisms. The following summary acknowledges that each country has unique underlying political and cultural factors that have influenced its response to the use of market mechanisms in the provision of health care. Those political and cultural influences are not going to be discussed in detail. Rather, the health care systems of various countries are going to be summarized in general terms in order to draw some conclusions for the purposes of enhancing the debate.[194]

Market Acceptors. The United States is the leading advocate of market mechanisms in the world. Because the health care system in the United States has been covered at length already, no further details are needed in this section. Other countries considered market acceptors, though, are Vietnam, Chile, Argentina, and Brazil.

Market Rejectors. These countries have a history of rejecting market mechanisms in health care, although they do accept some limited role of the market in their economic systems. They provide universal national health care for all of their residents. Market rejectors include Canada, Denmark, Sweden, the United Kingdom, Italy, and Belgium.

Canada is a prime example of a market rejector. The Canadian health care system is often compared to that of the United States to highlight the differences.[195] In 1984 the Canada Health Act passed, bringing universal health care to the nation. The Canadian provinces pay for 92 percent of hospital payments and 98.5 percent of physician reimbursements.[196] The health services are funded through a mixture of federal, provincial, and municipal taxes paid by individuals and corporations. There are also employer payroll taxes, premium payments made by individuals in certain provinces, and out-of-pocket monies—all of which help pay for the system.

Some services, such as outpatient prescription drugs and home health care, are not included in the Canadian Health Act. These services are provided at the discretion of the provinces, and most of them are provided for only the poor and elderly.[197] Unlike many other countries, Canada does not have private health insurance. Private insurance for coverage of the physician and hospital services that the provinces already provide is either outright prohibited or so restricted that it would not be economical to offer. It is available, however, for coverage of goods and services not provided for by the provinces, such as prescription drugs, dental work, and optometry. Approximately two-thirds of the country's population has some type of supplemental private insurance, which is often subsidized by employers as part of a benefit package.[198]

The Canadian system is described as ideal by many. In 2001 Canada spent 9.7 percent of its GDP on health care. Still, there are waiting lists for procedures, a shortage of both nurses and doctors, and a shortage of diagnostic technologies, such as computed tomography (CT) scanners and MRIs. Despite all the difficulties, Canada has managed to avoid the expansion of private insurance into its health care system.

Market Accommodators. These countries use some market practices and have a generally favorable attitude toward them. These countries also have strong histories of values of solidarity and universal access to health care, however, which they want to retain.[199] Two such countries are Switzerland and Australia, which were discussed earlier in the chapter. Other examples are Germany, France, Belgium, and The Netherlands.

Second-Thought Countries. These countries relied heavily on the market at one time but then became disillusioned with it. Because no country from this group has been discussed yet, let's look at New Zealand and the Czech Republic.

New Zealand had a single-payer tax-based universal health care program until rising costs and poor administration in the 1970s created problems for the system. In 1993 a set of reforms were adopted that used market mechanisms, such as higher user fees and a withdrawal of many government subsidies. These reforms did not work well. Competition did not develop smoothly, and efficiency was impeded, rather than enhanced. After 1996 many of the market mechanisms in these reforms were dropped. Still, the public in New Zealand wants a more efficient health care system, and there remains a powerful group of market proponents in government.[200]

The Czech Republic is another nation that tried market mechanisms in health care and then became disillusioned with them. While under communist control, the country had a tax-based universal health care system. However, the GDP devoted to health care was very low (4.1 percent in 1989).[201] With the revolution in 1989, the health care system underwent a major change. Market tactics were embraced. For example, a government health care proposal called for the decentralization of health care, for competitive services, and for consumer choice of health care provider.[202] During 1991 and 1992, health care facilities other than hospitals were privatized, and physicians were allowed to use a fee-for-service payment system, which promoted private medical practices. Several problems resulted from these changes, though. Between 1995 and 1996 the public insurance companies incurred heavy debts and became insolvent. Many hospitals could not pay for pharmaceuticals. So, in 1998 the Czech government stopped many of the market practices that had been adopted. Today health care is universal and free for all citizens.

Yet, some market practices still exist in the Czech Republic. Physicians are allowed to set up private practices. Patients are theoretically allowed to choose their health providers and hospitals, although in reality there are obstacles that discourage this. Although there are no private health insurance companies, people are allowed to purchase supplementary benefits from the public insurance funds. Also, 7.1 percent of the GDP is now going toward health care. Yet, there are many complaints about the system, and many people, particularly the younger generation, are advocating more market mechanisms.[203]

Country Comparisons. What does all of this tell us about the use of market mechanisms in the provision of health care? Callahan and Wasunna put several classes of health statistics into comparative tables to make some conclusions about health outcomes among the four categories of countries.

One table examines the gross domestic product per capita and health care expenditures in various countries. The GDP in the United States is far higher than any other nation in the world. The United States also spends more of its GDP on health care than any other country. Between 1970 and 2001 that amount rose over 50 percent, to $4,370 per person. In 2004 the United States spent 15 per cent of its GDP on health care.

In Europe the numbers are smaller but still high. For example, Switzerland spent over 10 percent of its GDP on health care. In fact, one of the lowest rates in Europe is in the Czech Republic, which spent just over 7 percent of its GDP on health care.[204]

Other Callahan and Wasunna tables reflect the wide variations between the United States and Europe regarding availability and use of diagnostic technologies and the numbers of hospital beds and physicians. The United States has the second largest number of MRI units per million people; only Switzerland has more. Several countries exceed the United States in CT scanners per million people. It is interesting to note that except for Italy, there is a negative correlation between the use of MRIs and CT scanners and the percentage of GDP devoted to health care expenditures.[205] The United States has one of the lowest ratios of physicians, 260 per 100,000 people, while of the European countries, Italy has the highest, with 567 physicians per 100,000 people. The United States has more average annual physician consultations per capita, at 8.9, than any European country. Even with all of its physicians, Italy only has 6.1 consultations per capita.[206] There is a large gap between the United States and European countries when analyzing the numbers of bypass and angioplasty procedures. The United States uses these procedures about three times as often per thousand people as any European country except for Belgium. Still, the average length of stay in the hospital for acute myocardial infractions is much shorter in the United States than in the European countries.[207]

Finally, statistics show that life expectancy at birth in the United States is shorter than in several European countries. At the age of sixty-five years, however, the United States begins to catch up with Europe for further life expectancy. After the age of eighty, life expectancy in the United States is the same as in Canada—and the highest in the world.[208] Callahan and Wasunna note that in the United States, at the age of sixty-five, people begin being covered by the federal Medicare program, which is a tax-financed system.[209]

Even with such comparisons, it is difficult to conclude whether one health care system is better than another. Each country has its own unique culture, history, political system, and population, which affect both its health care goals and the means used to achieve these goals. Thomas Rice notes that "different countries emphasize different objectives," which makes it difficult to conclude that one country has a better health care system than another.[210] Nonetheless, Callahan and Wasunna make a very good point when they state that "no country, or its politicians, seem to think—or at least would be willing to say—that a health care system with great health disparities between the rich and poor is a good arrangement, or that significant differences in access are beneficial for their citizens, or that gross inefficiency and its attendant poor quality care and high costs is an acceptable state of affairs."[211]

With the core principles of justice set forth in chapter 1, which represent criteria for evaluating whether any type of system is just, Catholic social thought cannot tolerate a health care system with large disparities. Although all countries use some combination of government and the market to fund and organize their health care systems, the United States relies the most on market mechanisms. And when examining major elements of a health care system, such as cost, health status, and access, the United States does not fare nearly as well as the European systems. The only seemingly important category in which the United States leads other nations is in the health status of people over the age of eighty. To repeat: This statistic can be directly traced to the superior health care available to them through the federal Medicare program.[212]

Still, one cannot dismiss the strong historical ties and deep roots that market practices have in the United States. It is unimaginable that they could fall out of favor in the near future. With this fact in mind, is it possible to reform the predominantly market-based system of the United States in a way that will fulfill, or at least come close to fulfilling, Catholic social teaching's requirements of justice? I will try to answer this question in the next chapter by using the Catholic justice tradition to evaluate the health care plans of four market proponents.

Notes

1. Callahan and Wasunna, *Medicine and the Market*, 37.
2. Peterson, "Introduction: Health Care," 11.
3. Callahan and Wasunna, *Medicine and the Market*, 20.
4. Ibid., 21.
5. For a good description of the project and possible consequences, see *Economist*, "Survey of the Human Genome."
6. Centers for Disease Control and Prevention, *National Vital Statistics*, 125.
7. Guyer et al., "Annual Summary of Vital Statistics," 1312.
8. Callahan and Wasunna, *Medicine and the Market*, 22.
9. Ibid., 22–23.
10. Starr, *Social Transformation of American Medicine*, 339.
11. For a good historical summary, see Rothstein, "Pharmaceuticals and Public Policy."
12. Callahan, *What Price Better Health?* 202–3.
13. Ibid., 203.
14. International Market Services, *I.M.S. Retail Drug Monitor*.
15. Starr, *Social Transformation of American Medicine*, 219.
16. Ibid.
17. Ibid., 116–19.
18. Ibid., 338–39.
19. Ibid., 340–41.
20. Ibid., 341.
21. Ibid., 342.
22. Ibid., 348.
23. Ibid.
24. Ibid., 352–63.

25. E. Richard Brown, "Public Policies to Extend Health Care Coverage," 37.

26. Starr, *Social Transformation of American Medicine*, 384.

27. Ibid.

28. Ibid.

29. Ibid., 396–97.

30. Sherman, "Health Care Spending Hits Record," A5.

31. Catholic Health Association of the United States, "Health Care in America," 1.

32. Callahan and Wasunna, *Medicine and the Market*, 228.

33. Kaiser Commission, *Health Care in America*, 10.

34. McGinley and Lueck, "Behind Drug-Benefit Debate," 1.

35. Ibid.

36. Copleston, *History of Philosophy*, 1–50.

37. Rice, *Economics of Health Reconsidered*, 174.

38. Ibid., 14.

39. Ibid., 18.

40. Gaynor and Vogt, "What Does Economics Have to Say?" 477.

41. Rice, *Economics of Health Reconsidered*, 67.

42. Ibid.

43. Ibid., 69.

44. Ibid.

45. Ibid., 74.

46. Hunt and Sherman, *Economics: An Introduction*, 212.

47. Ibid., 215.

48. Ibid., 216.

49. Rice, *Economics of Health Reconsidered*, 130.

50. Ibid., 132.

51. Hunt and Sherman, *Economics: An Introduction*, 252.

52. Ibid., 253.

53. Rice, *Economics of Health Reconsidered*, 81.

54. Ibid., 143.

55. Ibid., 203.

56. Ibid., 204.

57. Ibid., 24–25.

58. Ibid., 25.

59. Ibid., 148.

60. For a detailed analysis of market versus government failure, see Wolf, *Markets or Governments*.

61. Rice, *Economics of Health Reconsidered*, 206–7.

62. Arrow, "Uncertainty and the Welfare Economics."

63. See, for example, Folland et al., *Economics of Health*.

64. Arrow, "Uncertainty and the Welfare Economics," 941.

65. Ibid., 948–49.

66. Ibid., 949–50.

67. Ibid., 950.

68. Ibid., 951.

69. Ibid., 952.

70. Ibid.

71. Ibid., 953.

72. Ibid., 967.

73. Rice, *Economics of Health Reconsidered*, 24.

74. Ibid., 26.

75. Ibid., 37.

76. Ibid., 39–42.

77. Ibid., 56.

78. Ibid., 38.

79. Ibid., 43.

80. Ibid., 48.

81. Ibid.

82. Ibid., 49.

83. Ibid., 63.

84. Ibid., 63–64.

85. Ibid., 79.

86. Ibid., 85.

87. Ibid., 86.

88. Ibid., 87–88.

89. Ibid., 92.

90. Ibid.

91. Sen, *Choice, Welfare, and Measurement*, 94.

92. Rice, *Economics of Health Reconsidered*, 95.

93. Ibid., 96.

94. Ibid., 96–97.

95. Taylor, "What Price For-Profit Hospitals?" 1418.

96. Rice, *Economics of Health Reconsidered*, 147.

97. Ibid., 148.

98. Ibid., 149.

99. Ibid., 150.

100. Ibid., 190–92.

101. Ibid., 272.

102. Gaynor and Vogt, "What Does Economics Have to Say?" 476.

103. Ibid., 477.

104. Ibid.

105. Ibid., 477–78.

106. Ibid.

107. Ibid., 478.

108. Ibid., 479.

109. Ibid.

110. Ibid.

111. Ibid., 480.

112. Ibid., 481.

113. Ibid., 482–83.

114. Ibid., 484.

115. Ibid., 485.

116. Ibid.

117. Callahan and Wasunna, *Medicine and the Market*, 217.

118. Ibid., 217–18.

119. See, for example, Perez-Stable, "Managed Care Arrives in Latin America."

120. Starr, *Social Transformation of American Medicine*, 295–98.

121. Ibid., 333.

122. Committee on the Consequences of Uninsurance, *A Shared Destiny*, 37.

123. Starr, *Social Transformation of American Medicine*, 298.

124. Ibid., 328.

125. Ibid., 334.

126. Committee on the Consequences of Uninsurance, *A Shared Destiny*, 37.

127. Committee on the Consequences of Uninsurance, *Hidden Costs, Value Lost*, 42.

128. Gabel et al., "Health Benefits in 2003," 117.

129. Ibid., 119.

130. Rice, *Economics of Health Reconsidered*, 295–96.

131. Callahan and Wasunna, *Medicine and the Market*, 231.

132. Rice, *Economics of Health Reconsidered*, 276.

133. Ibid.

134. Wilcox, "Promoting Private Health Insurance in Australia," 152–62.

135. Ibid.

136. Wilcox, "Promoting Private Health Insurance in Australia."

137. Ibid.

138. Rice, *Economics of Health Reconsidered*, 216–19.

139. Gabel et al., "Health Benefits in 2003," 117.

140. Callahan and Wasunna, *Medicine and the Market*, 70.

141. Murray, "Balancing Values, Funding and Americanization of Expectations," 95.

142. Kominski and Melnick, "Managed Care and the Growth of Competition," 389–90.

143. Devettere, *Practical Decision Making*, 599–600.

144. *Health Maintenance Organizations Act.*

145. Kaiser Family Foundation, *Trends and Indicators, 2002,* 57.

146. I am using the models described in Devettere, *Practical Decision Making,* 599–600.

147. Milio, *Public Health in the Market,* 39.

148. Kaiser Family Foundation, *Employer Health Benefits Survey 2003,* 71.

149. *Aetna Health Inc., fka Aetna U.S., Healthcare Inc., et al. v. Davila.*

150. Goldstein, "For Patients' Rights," A4.

151. Kominski and Melnick, "Managed Care and the Growth of Competition," 392, 399.

152. Devettere, *Practical Decision Making,* 601.

153. Kaiser Family Foundation, *Trends and Indicators, 2004 Update,* Exhibit 3:4.

154. Kaiser Family Foundation, *Employer Health Benefits Survey 2003,* 183.

155. Enthoven, "Employment-Based Health Insurance," 238.

156. Callahan and Wasunna, *Medicine and the Market,* 211.

157. Ibid., 211–12.

158. Saltman and Figueras, *European Health Care Reform.*

159. Callahan and Wasunna, *Medicine and the Market,* 213.

160. Kaiser Family Foundation, *Employee Health Benefits: 2004 Annual Survey,* 4.

161. Ibid.

162. Ibid., ch. 6, p. 7.

163. Callahan and Wasunna, *Medicine and the Market,* 213.

164. Ibid., 214.

165. Ibid.

166. Ibid., 215.

167. Ibid.

168. Ibid., 216.

169. Ibid.

170. Ibid.

171. Ibid.

172. Ibid.

173. Devettere, *Practical Decision Making,* 596.

174. For a good overview of physician compensation, see Christensen, "Ethically Important Distinctions"; Orentlicher, "Paying Physicians More to Do Less."

175. Callahan and Wasunna, *Medicine and the Market,* 225.

176. Ibid., 225–26.

177. Managed Health Care Improvement Task Force, *Financial Incentives for Providers,* 74.

178. Ibid., 79.

179. Callahan and Wasunna, *Medicine and the Market,* 226.

180. Ibid.

181. Ibid.

182. For a good, concise discussion of this issue, see Orentlicher, *Paying Physicians More to Do Less*, 161–62.

183. Callahan and Wasunna, *Medicine and the Market*, 227.

184. Baldwin, "Unsocializing Medicine," 24.

185. Callahan and Wasunna, *Medicine and the Market*, 223.

186. Ron Lieber, "Health Savings Plan You Can't Get."

187. Ibid.

188. Ibid.

189. Ibid.

190. Callahan and Wasunna, *Medicine and the Market*, 223.

191. Ibid.

192. Ibid., 224.

193. Ibid., 225.

194. I am using typologies from ibid., 91–93.

195. For a concise history of Canadian health care, see Murray, "Balancing Values, Funding and Americanization of Expectations."

196. Rice, *Economics of Health Reconsidered*, 280.

197. Ibid.

198. Ibid.

199. For an excellent discussion of solidarity values, see Callahan and Wasunna, *Medicine and the Market*, 90–1.

200. Ibid., 107–8.

201. Ibid., 106.

202. Ibid.

203. Ibid., 107.

204. Ibid., 231.

205. Ibid.

206. Ibid., 233.

207. Ibid., 232.

208. Ibid., 229.

209. Ibid., 228.

210. Rice, *Economics of Health Reconsidered*, 270.

211. Callahan and Wasunna, *Medicine and the Market*, 233–34.

212. Ibid., 235.

4

The Market Organization
Approach to Health Care

The inner workings of the way health care is organized and managed are the focus of the market organization approach. The aim of this approach is not to reflect on, challenge, or change the underlying values that drive the health care system. Rather, it is to change the way those values are utilized. One of the primary goals of this approach is to address how market practices can produce a better and more efficient system than government can.

The market organization approach emphasizes profit, private enterprise, and competition. It uses incentives to promote cost effectiveness and legal contracts to establish relationships between insurers and the insured, between insurers and providers, and often between purchasers and providers. This approach promotes for-profit institutions as health care providers and emphasizes a system where, although some federal and state regulations exist, most of the decisions about insurance products and the distribution of health care are made by private actors.[1]

This chapter examines the work of four secular economists who promote their own plans to organize health care by using market tactics—Milton Friedman, Regina Herzlinger, Mark Pauly, and Alain Enthoven—chosen specifically because they represent the spectrum of market thinking. It is important to note that they are all Americans and, as a practical matter, none of their plans has completely triumphed. (Still, no single system has triumphed anywhere, anyway.)

Although Catholic social thought would find problems with all four economic approaches, they also have their positive elements. I will first review the plan of each thinker, and then I analyze it in light of Catholic social thought. I conclude with some general thoughts on how the market organization approach could perhaps be made more harmonious with Catholic social thought.

Milton Friedman: A Market Purist's Cure for Health Care

To understand the impact that widely acclaimed Nobel laureate Milton Friedman has had on economics, a short review of U.S. economics before Friedman will be helpful. Then I will review Friedman's anthropology, which is foundational to his economic theories and has in fact had great influence on the theories of most market proponents. Next will come an examination of Friedman's proposal to help solve the nation's health care problems. Finally, I will assess Friedman's proposal for compatibility with Catholic social thought.

The House That Keynes Built

Up until the mid-1970s, the economic thought of John Maynard Keynes reigned supreme in the United States and Great Britain. Keynes (1883–1946) is often regarded as "the intellectual godfather of postwar welfare capitalism."[2] In the 1930s, while the world suffered an immense economic depression, many saw capitalism as a failure and began to embrace socialism. Keynes's 1936 book, *General Theory of Employment, Interest, and Money*, took aim at the laissez-faire approach to economic policy, taking on Adam Smith and his concept that an economy could self-regulate. Keynes thought that the depression was "a product of the mistaken assumption that the market would bring about full employment on its own."[3] He tried to show what had happened to the capitalistic economy to cause the depression, so that capitalism could be saved.

Keynes's theory is too complex to go into much detail here. In short, Keynes developed new theories regarding the process of production and income-expenditure flow. He concluded that the major cause of the depression was the inability of capitalists to locate sufficient investment opportunities to offset the rising levels of savings generated by economic growth.[4] Keynes's unique contribution was to envision how the relationship between savings and income could lead to a stable, albeit depressed, level of income with large rates of unemployment.[5] His solution was that government should step in when savings exceeded investment, borrow the excess savings, and spend the money on social programs. The spending by government would increase the amount of money put into the spending stream and then create full-employment equilibrium.[6] In other words, Keynes provided a rationale for governments to increase spending to fight off high rates of unemployment. He believed, in the words of Jerry Muller, that government must compensate for "the errors created by avarice, usury, and a debased culture that made individuals too frugal and prone to defer gratification."[7]

Keynes went on to become one of the most influential economists in the Western world. By the 1950s Keynesian macroeconomics, his take on the behavior of the aggregate economy, was well-established public policy. Since World War II, governments had used Keynes's theories and fought unemployment with increased government spending or an increase in the money supply. These policies caused inflation but could usually be controlled by decreasing the money supply. Runaway inflation and high unemployment marked the 1960s and early 1970s, though.

By the mid-1970s, these problems became much worse. Keynesian policies seemed no longer effective, as the nation experienced stagflation, a combination of both unemployment and inflation.[8] The situation called for new government economic policies. One of the people responsible for an injection of new policies was Milton Friedman.

The Market That Friedman Built

Milton Friedman was one of "the Chicago boys." As with many other universities, the University of Chicago's famous economics faculty came together in the 1930s and 1940s with a combination of distinguished academics, new academic stars, and European academics, some of whom were fleeing fascism.[9] By the end of the 1950s, the "Chicago School" had emerged. Known as supporters of laissez-faire capitalism and opponents to Keynesian economic theory, the Chicago School gained a reputation for rigorous academics and an allegiance to the market.[10]

In 1946 Friedman became an economics professor at Chicago. He vigorously attacked Keynesian economics and enthusiastically promoted free markets, seeing "a direct, explicit, and unabashed connection between capitalism and democracy."[11] Friedman argued for a balanced federal budget, a natural rate of unemployment, and a "strict monetary rule," whereby the Federal Reserve should not intervene in the money supply at all. In 1976 the Royal Swedish Academy of Sciences awarded him its Prize in Economics.[12] By the 1980s several of his theories had become widely accepted into mainstream economic theory.

Friedman was unabashedly in favor of free markets. He once wrote, "Fundamentally, there are two ways of coordinating the economic activities of millions. One is central direction involving the use of coercion—the technique of

the army and the modern totalitarian state. The other is the voluntary cooperation of individuals—the technique of the marketplace."[13] Friedman was
not a health care economist per se and in fact wrote very little on health care.
However, what he *did* write is considered important and influential. Moreover,
because he was one of the most prominent economic thinkers of the second
half of the twentieth century, his arguments about the market in health care
bear a thorough investigation.

Before examining Friedman's position on health care, though, I am going
to analyze some of the foundational economic tenets that implicitly influence
his thoughts on health care. In 1962 he published his classic book on economics
Capitalism and Freedom, which sets forth his basic anthropology: Freedom is the
ultimate and most cherished value; freedom is to be preserved and expanded.[14]
Friedman equates economic freedom with political freedom, which he defines
as "the absence of coercion of a man by his fellow men."[15] He goes on to suggest
that, given this fact, the ultimate threat to political freedom is coercion. The
power to coerce is the most fundamental peril to freedom, and government
has this power.[16] A government—or political authority, as he sometimes calls
it—"can never duplicate the variety and diversity of individual action" and must
be limited, must be dispersed.[17]

Friedman sees the market as a mechanism that reduces the issues that must
be regulated by government, minimizing the extent to which government needs
to be involved in the lives of its citizens. He does not advocate the elimination
of government. Rather, he recognizes that government in a "free society" is vital
for "determining the 'rules of the game'" and to act "as an umpire to interpret
and enforce the rules decided on";[18] that is, to maintain law and order, define
property rights and other rules of economics, adjudicate disputes about the
interpretation of these rights and economic rules, enforce contracts, provide a
monetary system, counter "true" monopolies, and work with private charities to
protect children and care for the mentally incompetent.[19]

A good example of Friedman's ideology at work is found in his response
to the bishops' 1986 pastoral letter, *Economic Justice for All*. Friedman attacks
the letter on several grounds. With his dislike of government, Friedman naturally criticizes the bishops' reliance on government. He argues that they do not
advocate voluntary associations to rectify economic woes, but instead call for
government to take certain actions to remedy injustices.

Friedman reviews the major objectives of the pastoral letter and critiques
them individually. He begins with the bishops' call for government to make a
major commitment to achieve full employment. Friedman contends that after

World War II several European nations, such as Great Britain and France, adopted a commitment to full employment through policies similar to those advocated by the bishops. He contends that these policies failed miserably and resulted in very high unemployment rates in the countries that tried them. Moreover, he attributes the stagflation of the 1960s and 1970s to the same economic policies touted by the bishops. Friedman argues that since the 1970s, many European countries have changed their economic policies and moved away from government involvement and toward a free market approach. With the free market approach, Friedman contends, came both greater employment (more jobs) and lower unemployment rates (a smaller proportion of the population actively looking for work). He concludes that "experience clearly provides no support for the idea that a government declaration of a policy of full employment is an effective device for eliminating unemployment."[20]

Friedman is also critical of the bishops' objective of fostering greater economic opportunities for the poor through government intervention. Again, Friedman argues that all of the policies recommended by the bishops, such as job training, apprenticeships, and fiscal and monetary policies, have been tried, but to no avail. For Friedman the free market is the best way to help the poor. "The most effective engine for improving the lot of the poor, the one method that has enabled low-income people to rise on the scale to become middle-income people, has been a free capitalist system and a free market."[21]

He backs up this statement with the following historical argument. Many people who are reading his work are descendended from immigrants who left the lands of their birth to come to the United States with very little in terms of possessions or financial assets. The nineteenth and early twentieth centuries were times of great progress, and the immigrant families were able to make better lives for themselves and their families without any government assistance or government programs. He concludes that "if today's government programs had existed, it would have been impossible for many of our forebears to have emigrated to the United States. We are the products of what people seeking to improve their lot can achieve themselves through voluntary cooperation in a free market."[22] Friedman compares countries to reinforce this point. He contends that a comparison of the former East Germany with West Germany, and Red China with Hong Kong, shows that free markets and capitalism markedly improved the conditions of the poor.[23]

Moreover, Friedman actually names government as one of the major causes of poverty: "Government policies are the major source of the residual poverty in the United States."[24] He gives the following examples of harmful government policies and programs and why they are defective: minimum wage laws, which actually raise the unemployment rate among teenagers; a poor public education system, which does not adequately train black youths; urban renewal and public housing, which have become filled with families without fathers and therefore provide no good male role models for children; and government support of trade unions that discourage minority membership because it is not in the self-interest of the people who are already members.[25] Friedman goes on to argue, using information from Charles Murray's *Losing Ground*, that the Great Society programs started during President Lyndon Johnson's administration (1963–69), with great hopes for winning the "War on Poverty," actually caused the rates of poverty, crime, and family breakups to increase, rather than to decrease.[26]

The final objective of the bishops that Friedman challenges is their goal to improve the conditions of the poor in foreign countries through foreign aid and foreign investments. He claims that such policies must not be helpful, because "the countries that have received the largest amount of foreign aid have had the least success in improving the lot of their people."[27] He contends that foreign aid merely empowers the foreign governments to whom it is given and that most underdeveloped countries have "tyrannical governments that are running them in the interest of the governing class and not of the people."[28] His solution to poverty in developing countries is that they open their markets to foreign investments and encourage free markets.

Friedman also takes issue with what he calls the "collectivist moral vision" of the bishops' letter. Here he is referring to the bishops' contention that a society and a government have moral obligations. Friedman presents the alternative moral view that "a 'society' is a collection of individuals; that the basic entity is the individual or, more fundamentally, the family, and that only individuals can have moral obligations."[29] Only people, therefore, can have moral obligations and duties, and government is merely the means by which people cooperate to achieve common ends. His objection to a collectivist moral vision is particularly strong when he critiques the bishops' notion of economic rights, specifically their characterization of putting economic rights on a par with civil and political rights. Friedman maintains that there can be no right to adequate nutrition, because such a right cannot be enjoyed by everyone simultaneously in the way the right to free speech can, for example, unless "there is some cornucopia from which the food comes."[30] He acknowledges that the bishops do indeed list some "true economic rights," such as a right to own property, which everyone can enjoy at the same time. But a right to "food, housing, adequate nutrition and the like . . . reflects a collectivist moral vision that is wholly inconsistent" with the Church's designation of human dignity as the standard against which economic life should be measured.[31]

The little Friedman wrote on health care reflected his love of the market and disdain of government. His first endeavor into the field of health care economics was an editorial called "Gammon's Law Points to Health-Care Solution," published in the *Wall Street Journal* in 1991. He then expanded the editorial into an article published by the prominent public policy journal *The Public Interest* in 2001.[32] The article, "How to Cure Health Care," attempts to analyze why health care costs are so high in the United States and to make recommendations to solve this problem. He begins his essay by arguing that the provision of medicine in developed countries has displayed three major features since World War II: rapid advancement in the science of medicine, large increases in spending on medical care, and increasing dissatisfaction with the delivery of medical care by both its consumers and its suppliers.[33] Friedman goes on to assert that the key difference between advancements in medicine and advancements in other kinds of technology, such as communications and transportation, is the role of government. Friedman claims that with technological advances other than in medicine, the strategy, funding, production, and distribution are primarily done through private avenues. When it comes to medical care, though, government has played a major role in its financing, production, and distribution.

As evidence to support his claim, Friedman notes that "direct government spending on health exceeds 75 percent of total health spending for 15 OECD [Organization for Economic Co-operation and Development, its members thirty basically highly industrialized democracies] countries. . . . For the United States, such subsidization raises the fraction of health care spending financed directly or indirectly by the government to over 50 percent."[34] He then asks, What are countries receiving in return for the money they are putting into health care? Friedman argues that it is difficult to answer this question, because it is nearly impossible to measure the output, or the outcome, of the spending. He examines various possible ways of measuring health outputs, such as number of beds occupied or life expectancy at birth. However, he finds these measurements inadequate because they do not actually reflect what it means to be in "good health," nor do they allow for other factors, such as the quantity and quality of food and water available to the measured population, which may influence the statistics.

Nonetheless, Friedman notes that there is one statistic that is indisputable: The United States spends more of its GDP on health care than any other nation. There are two reasons, according to Friedman, that explain this fact. First, most payments made to physicians come not directly from the patients' own finances but from a third party, such as an insurance company or government. Friedman suggests that medical costs, unlike food or gasoline, are paid for by third parties because they are exempt from income tax only if they are provided for by the employer. In other words, if an employee pays directly for medical care with his or her own money, the amount comes out of his or her income after income tax. If an employer pays for the medical expenses through the provision of health insurance, though, the costs to the employer are treated as a tax-deductible expense for the employer.[35] Moreover, with the passage of Medicare and Medicaid, government became a third-party payer. Friedman finds fault with this system and asks why we single out health care when other things, such as food, would not be tax-exempt if paid for by an employer.[36] Friedman claims that third-party payment for medical care has the potential to be another example where "one bad government policy leads to another."[37]

Friedman argues that third-party payments have two important effects on medical care, both of which raise health care costs. First, they force employees to rely on their employers to arrange for their medical care. Second, it results in employees taking a higher percentage of their total remuneration in the form of medical care than they would if medical spending had the same tax status as other expenditures.[38]

Friedman also emphasizes that health insurance is very different from other types of insurance, which protects people against an event that is unlikely to occur but would involve large losses if it were to occur. For example, homeowner's insurance is purchased to protect the homeowner from financial disaster if the house should burn down. Yet, medical insurance is commonly relied upon to pay not just for unlikely disasters but "for regular medical examinations and often for prescriptions."[39]

He concludes that if the "tax exemption for employer-provided medical care and Medicare and Medicaid had never been enacted, the insurance market for medical care would probably have developed as other insurance markets have. The typical form of medical insurance would have been catastrophic insurance—i.e., insurance with a very high deductible."[40] Hence, Friedman contends third-party payments have led to the bureaucratization of medical care, whereby "a medical transaction is not simply between a caregiver and a patient" but has to be "approved as 'covered' by a bureaucrat and the appropriate payment authorized."[41]

Next Friedman discusses Gammon's Law, formulated by British physician Max Gammon after studying the British medical system. He proposed "the theory of bureaucratic displacement," which states that in "a bureaucratic system . . . *increase in expenditure* will be matched by *fall in production*. . . . Such systems will act rather like 'black holes,' in the economic universe, simultaneously sucking in resources, and shrinking in terms of 'emitted production.'"[42] Friedman argues that the medical system in the United States parallels that of Great Britain because "here too input has been going up sharply relative to output."[43] He concludes that "the high cost and inequitable character of our medical care system is the direct result of our steady movement toward reliance on third-party payment. A cure requires reversing course, that is, reprivatizing medical care by eliminating most third-party payment and restoring the role of insurance to providing protection against major medical catastrophes."[44]

Having made this conclusion, Friedman presents his "cure" for health care. He advocates the repeal of the tax-exempt status of employer-provided health care; the termination of Medicare and Medicaid; the deregulation of most insurance; and restricting the role of the federal government to taking care of the "hard cases," when it comes to financing health care.[45] He acknowledges that his recommendations are not politically feasible. Still, he argues that the health care system needs a "cure" and must be "reprivatized," with an emphasis on catastrophic coverage.[46]

The mechanism that fulfills Friedman's requirements for covering health care is the medical savings account (MSA). As noted in chapter 3, as part of the 2003 Medicare Reform Bill, MSAs were discontinued in January 2004 and replaced by the health savings account (HSA). Although HSAs were not in existence when Friedman wrote his article, I think it is fair to say he would support them, because they are so closely related to MSAs and accomplish many of the goals he advocated. They act primarily as catastrophic policies (major medical policies with a high deductible), they do not involve employer contributions, and they require participants to pay for their own routine medical care without any involvement of third-party payments until the deductible is met. Friedman contends that MSAs (or HSAs) are a great solution to the ills of the health care system:

This reform would solve the problem of the currently medically unin-sured, eliminate most of the bureaucratic structure, free medical practi-tioners from an increasingly heavy burden of paperwork and regulation, and lead many employers and employees to convert employer-provided medical care into a higher cash wage. The taxpayer would save money because total government costs would plummet. The family would be relieved of one of its major concerns—the possibility of being impover-ished by a major medical catastrophe—and most could readily finance the remaining medical costs.[47]

Catholic Social Thought and Milton Friedman's Plan

Milton Friedman's recommendations for health care are not very compatible with Catholic social thought. His ideology rests on the foundational belief that freedom, political and economic, is the ultimate value to be protected at all costs. Although Catholic social thought is no fan of socialism or communism, it recognizes most, if not all, of the traditional human rights encompassed in a democracy, such as the right to religious freedom, the right to assembly, and the right to free speech.[48] Yet, the bases for, and definitions of what constitutes, political and economic freedom in Catholic social thought differ greatly from Friedman's viewpoint.

For Friedman political and economic freedom is desirable because he sup-ports the rights of the *individual* person in the atomistic sense, as separate and disconnected beings. He does not perceive individuals in the social sense, or within a community, as the Church perceives them. Furthermore, for Friedman freedom means to be free *from* something—namely, from the coercion of other people. In Catholic social thought, political and economic freedom is defined within the context of freedom *for* something, as in the sense of having freedom to achieve full human dignity. Thus, in Catholic social thought political free-dom is highly desirable because it allows people the ability to develop fully as human beings, which means having the conditions necessary for this develop-ment, including the ability to participate in the institutions that bear on this.

Moreover, Friedman does not recognize any notion of the common good, which is the reason he vehemently criticizes what he calls the bishops' "collec-tivist moral vision." He does recognize that individuals may have common ends and that a purpose of government is to help achieve these common ends. Yet, common ends are very different from a common good. There is no morality associated with common ends. Common ends can be any agreed-upon goal. Hence, if a group of individuals agree that their goal in life is to make as much money as possible to spend on themselves, this would be their common end. There is no social obligation required of common ends. So, in Friedman's work, the sense of communal social obligation is completely absent. In Catholic social thought, on the other hand, the good of the entire community is more important than the good of the individual. Even though agreeing upon the goals of the common good can be difficult, it nevertheless promotes human dignity for all individuals, not just for some.

Another major difference between Friedman's thought and Catholic social teaching is the role government should play in people's lives. Friedman is very explicit in his disdain for government. His view of government's role is very similar to that of the social contract theorist John Locke. He sees government as necessary only to act as an umpire to oversee very minimal rules and regulations, such as those defining property rights, to provide a monetary system for its citizens, and to provide an adjudicator for disputes. In contrast, the Catholic Church sees the state, or government, as an essential element in service to the common good. The Church's attitude toward government is best summed up by John XXIII's statement that "the whole reason for the existence of civil authorities is the realization of the common good."[49] Thus, Catholic social thought views government in a much more positive light than Friedman. Still, with its support of subsidiarity and socialization, Catholic social thought does not advocate a totalitarian view that would allow government to dominate the family, local communities, and other forms of smaller human associations. Instead, Catholic social thought recognizes that government may be the best entity to "lead to an appropriate structuring of the human community."[50]

With these major differences between Friedman and Catholic social thought, it is not difficult to conclude that Friedman's cure for health care is clearly deficient for several reasons. There is no question that Friedman wants to find a solution to the serious problem of soaring health care costs, and this is admirable. Moreover, his observations about the contribution that third-party payments have made to escalating health care costs are well stated. So, too, is his criticism that the United States spends far too much of its GDP on health care.

However, his solution to these problems is inadequate. Whereas Catholic social thought perceives access to basic health care as a right, Friedman argues that it is not a right. He bases this claim on the concept that for something to be a "right," everyone must be able to enjoy it at the same time. Catholic social thought does not go this far. Since Leo XIII the Church has endorsed the notion that human rights exist. Claims regarding economic and other human rights based on natural rights theory are now understood by the Church as stemming from natural law. For example, *Pacem in terris* contains a list of human rights, including economic rights, based on natural law theory, which was expanded in *Guadium et spes*. Economic rights are seen as necessary to promote human dignity and the common good because "there must be made available to all men everything necessary for leading a life truly human."[51] Moreover, the specific right to sufficient health care is mentioned in several Church documents, including *Pacem in terris*, the bishops' pastoral letter on health care, and John Paul II's address to the 34th General Assembly of the United Nations on October 24, 1979.

Friedman's recommendation that MSAs (or their replacement, HSAs) should be a primary mechanism to help solve our health care woes is very problematic. First, there are deep concerns about how people with chronic conditions, such as diabetes, will fare with HSAs. One worry is that the chronically ill will drain their savings accounts year after year because they will continually pass the deductible.[52] Other critics of HSAs charge that high-deductible insurance policies will cause people, especially those with low incomes and less disposable income, to delay needed medical care because they will want to keep their money as long as possible.

Moreover, HSAs are designed to encourage the active involvement of individuals in their medical decisions, but critics argue that the average individual is not well equipped to decide what medical care is essential and what is not. In many instances, people do not have sufficient information to make good health care decisions that are also cost-containing decisions.[53] Finally, critics contend that MSAs/HSAs are relatively ineffective in controlling health care costs, because about 10 percent of people, often with chronic or multiple health problems, make up about 69 percent of overall health costs. These people will continue to have high health costs regardless of what incentives are presented to them to curb health care spending.[54]

Another major flaw in Friedman's cure for health care is that it simply does not address the needs of the poor and chronically ill. Catholic social thought teaches that we have a special obligation to the poor and vulnerable, but Friedman simply ignores their plight. His article emphasizes the rising expenditures on health care, but it does not address issues of access or distributive justice.

This is not surprising, because he does not believe people have a right to basic health care or that there should be a "just distribution" of health care.

Moreover, Friedman expressly advocates the elimination of Medicare and Medicaid. He readily admits that this is politically unacceptable, so he argues that a Medicare and Medicaid recipient should have the option of either keeping his or her federal benefits or acquiring an MSA (HSA). But nowhere in his proposal does he address the fact that there are millions of middle- and lower-income Americans, many who work full- or part-time, who neither qualify for Medicare or Medicaid nor have health insurance at all. Either Friedman assumes that such people can afford the high-deductible plan, or he does not care whether they have any plan at all. Regardless, too many people do not have the disposable income necessary to buy such a plan, nor can they afford to pay for health care until they meet the deductible and the actual insurance policy begins to pay out. The chronically ill are at a particular disadvantage with such a plan because they will continually drain their accounts each year.

Friedman's plan is not compatible with Catholic social thought. Although it is possible that HSAs might help control health care costs, which would promote the common good, they would benefit only people who have large disposable incomes and are relatively healthy. But they would provide less, rather than greater, access to health care; they do not benefit the poor and vulnerable; they circumvent any role for government; and they are directed solely at controlling the demand side of health care.

Regina Herzlinger: Consumer-Driven Health Care

Regina E. Herzlinger is the Nancy R. McPherson Professor of Business Administration Chair of the Harvard Business School, and the first woman to be tenured at the Harvard Business School. Although she does not refer directly to Milton Friedman, his influence can be seen in her work.

After President George W. Bush's 2004 State of the Union address, Herzlinger wrote, "Bravo! President Bush espoused free-market principles for health care in his State of the Union speech. After Hillary Clinton's bid for a centrally controlled system, it's great to have someone in office who understands that health care, like everything else in our economy, must follow market principles.... Sadly, the president's plans fall short of a real market-based health care system."[55] For Herzlinger "a real market-based health care system" is a consumer-driven health care system "that rewards productivity by empowering providers *and* consumers."[56] Consumer-driven health care is Herzlinger's answer to what she sees as the failure of managed care, which occurred, according to Herzlinger, because of limitations on physician and consumer choice, or because "it tried to supplant the judgment of consumers and providers with that of health insurance executives."[57]

Herzlinger has written several hundred pages advocating her consumer-driven health care plan. She calls it "the new solution."[58] In her 1997 book, *Market Driven Health Care: Who Wins, Who Loses in the Transformation of America's Largest Service Industry*, she describes how she developed the plan.[59] While she was writing her doctoral thesis, she worked at a neighborhood health center in a working-class town across the river from a large city. She noticed a huge disparity between the two in health care resources and the overall health of the residents, with the larger city coming out far ahead. She also noticed, over the course of the next several years, how certain companies, such as in the manufacturing sector, made several innovative changes in their organizational structures to save the town's industry. Herzlinger argues that changes in the use of technology, in what she calls "employee empowerment," and in employees' gaining greater access to information saved the industry.

Herzlinger also noticed that "these ideas seem to have eluded much of the health system. All too many health providers are instead busily replicating the mistakes of the long-gone manufacturing giants, consolidating a fragmented industry in the belief that 'big is beautiful' and implementing top-down directives for delivery of health care."[60] By 1986 she was convinced that the innovations that reshaped manufacturing could be used to reshape the health care system.

Herzlinger chose to espouse the use of the market, with its innovative and consumer-oriented approach, to save the health care system in the United States. She argues that the market, "not managed care, but a true market, the great organic confluence of consumers and providers that characterizes virtually every other sector of our economy—will provide the solution to the deep problems that plague the American health care system."[61]

For Herzlinger a consumer-driven health care system is one where patients are considered, and consider themselves, *consumers*. Furthermore, today there is a new breed of consumers in the United States: "They know what they want, they want it fast, and they want it when they want it."[62] This new generation of consumers is smart, assertive, and demands convenience. Yet, she claims the health care system in the United States does not cater to these qualities. It is burdensome, complicated, and very, very inconvenient, which denies Americans much-needed health care services and thereby diminishes productivity, particularly due to absenteeism.[63]

Herzlinger suggests that there are two main causes of this inconvenience: legal barriers and managerial barriers. Anticompetitive laws, as she calls them, are responsible for stifling innovation. Herzlinger cites the optometry industry as an example. In the 1970s it was very difficult for customers to get copies of their eye correction prescriptions, advertising for optical services was prohibited in many locales, and in many states optometrists were prevented from working for opticians or for chain eyewear stores. She argues that these regulations were serious impediments to competition. Once they were removed, the prices of eyewear dropped, while the quality has increased.[64]

Still, Herzlinger contends, even when there are no legal barriers to competition in the health industry, there are managerial barriers. Two health care providers illustrate her point. Health Stop was a health care clinic that was akin to a supermarket—"easy to reach and easy to use."[65] No appointments were necessary, and short waiting times were supposed to be the norm. But the waiting times were very long. Herzlinger attributes this to, among other things, the fact that Health Stop paid its physicians fixed salaries, rather than on a fee-for-service basis. This gave the physicians no incentive to see patients quickly or to delegate to the support staff in such a manner that would speed up services. Herzlinger argues that Health Stop could have taken a course of action to make certain that their doctors were sufficiently motivated, but its lack of knowledge and experience with the health care profession stymied its ability to solve its problems.

In sharp contrast to the Health Stop experience, Herzlinger presents the story of Dr. Bernard Salick. His daughter had cancer, and her long, arduous experience with the medical system taught her father some lessons in medical care management. Dr. Salick established his own cancer treatment services with a mind to avoid the pitfalls his daughter had fallen into during her treatment. His clinics specialize only in cancer treatment; maintain beautiful and comfortable facilities, which have a very pleasant ambience about them; provide social support for children and other relatives who might accompany a patient to treatment; and promote an active exchange of ideas among the medical specialists who staff them. Herzlinger quotes *The Economist*: "Salick has . . . become the world's first full-service disease management firm."[66]

For the health care system, Herzlinger advocates "mastery," which she defines as "the success of businesses that provide customers with information, choices, and a sense of control."[67] Moreover, there are several ways that consumers themselves can be encouraged to "master their health," such as through becoming better educated about medical issues, perhaps by conducting informal research (even just "looking it up"), and through using such health aids as vitamins and exercise equipment.[68] A health care system can also provide mastery in other ways, such as identifying the parts of the health care system that already are convenient, reasonably priced, and filled with information. Herzlinger claims that such products are found "where health care products are paid for directly by consumers, such as eyewear or information on self-care."[69] She also mentions the internet and national magazines as excellent sources for health care information.[70]

Mastery also means guaranteeing that we retain "what is good about our health care—choice, technology, control, and convenience."[71] Herzlinger then proceeds to examine what she calls three types of "diets" that are used, to various degrees of success, to trim "not only overweight people, but large government entities and a jumbo American health care system."[72] She begins with the downsizing diet, which involves across-the-board cuts, layoffs, and other methods seen as cost saving, such as HMOs. However, Herzlinger claims, HMOs actually save money by rationing health care, by providing fewer resources. This, she argues, reduces the quality of care and discriminates against the sick.[73]

Herzlinger's second diet is called the upsizing, or "big is beautiful," diet. In the health care arena this diet manifests itself in mergers. Herzlinger notes that in the 1990s there was a trend to merge in the health care industry. For example, in 1994, 650 hospitals merged.[74] Numerous managed-care organizations also merged in the mid-nineties, so that by 1996 seven HMOs accounted for 74 percent of all enrollments.[75] The merger trend also affected medical suppliers, such as pharmaceutical manufacturers and producers of medical technology.[76]

Herzlinger explains that mergers can take place through horizontal or vertical integration, either of which can greatly expand a health care organization. Horizontal integration occurs when a health care entity purchases several hospitals, nursing homes, and/or physician practices, creating a chain of integrated health care systems. One example is Columbia Health Care Corporation. Formed in 1987, Columbia had a chain of 326 hospitals with revenues of $17.6 billion by 1995. Due to its large size, Columbia had tremendous bidding power for equipment and services, which initially saved millions of dollars. This was because when similar types of organizations merge, duplicated expenses are eliminated, and "best demonstrated practices" replicated, throughout the integrated system.[77] However, Herzlinger suggests that upon stricter scrutiny, horizontally integrated systems are neither more efficient nor more cost-effective than their smaller counterparts.[78]

With vertical integration, health care organizations are reorganized so that all health care services, including physician practices, surgery centers, pharmacies, and insurers, are owned and managed under one integrated system. Theoretically, such an organization would provide patients with whatever care they needed and would lower costs. Kaiser Permanente is an example of a vertically integrated organization. But such health care systems also had problems. Herzlinger looks at vertically integrated companies in other industries, like IBM and General Motors, and argues that large layoffs and questions about their ability to provide internal suppliers are evidence of cracks in the armor of vertical integration.[79] She suggests that the major reason vertical integration does not work well is that when markets are dominated by large firms, there is little competition with pricing, while at the same time a tremendous use of marketing tries to gain artificial competitive advantages. In her words, "Large providers can distort perfect markets."[80] Small, innovative firms are essential to creating a market that promotes price competition. Herzlinger cites reports in *Modern Healthcare* to give several examples of vertically integrated health care systems that are experiencing financial problems.[81] She concludes her analysis of vertical integration by stating that "in the end, in a mature industry, vertical integration fails primarily for one reason: It is very hard to implement."[82]

Because managed care, integration, downsizing, and upsizing all fail to solve the woes of the health care system, Herzlinger recommends her third "diet" for health care, which she calls "resizing." It is based on the concept of the focused factory. In a 1974 issue of *Harvard Business Review*, Wickham Skinner's "Focused Factory" argued that America's productivity crisis was caused by complex and overly broad factories.[83] He urged that a company learn to focus on a concise, manageable group of products; restructure manufacturing policies to focus on one express objective; and view efficiency problems as affecting the whole manufacturing process, not merely the efficiency of the workforce. Herzlinger sums up Skinner's research by repeating his conclusion that "simplicity and repetition breed competence."[84]

With Skinner's research in mind, Herzlinger advocates using the "focused factory" in health care, as characterized by the following. It is "a multidisciplinary group of people who work together to achieve a clear, limited objective."[85] They should not be organized according to physician specialties but according to requirements of the patients, because focused health care factories "*always* contain *all* the resources needed to provide for a patient."[86] For example, a cancer-focused factory provides total care for its cancer patients. It is not just a specialty clinic filled with oncologists. Rather, it also provides care for problems that accompany cancer, such as anemia. It provides diagnosis, treatment, and psychotherapy as well as hospital, outpatient, and in-home care. Focused factories can be located in local satellite units, and "a relatively small number . . . targeted at a handful of high-cost diseases, and at the relatively few severely ill patients with them, could provide enormous benefits."[87]

Yet, according to Herzlinger, there is one major problem preventing the adoption of the focused factory model: "Under the present fragmented insurance reimbursement system, health care–focused factories are not economically feasible."[88] Her solution is a consumer-driven health care system. Consumer-driven health care requires that all employees have the two Cs and one I: "Substantially greater *choice* of highly differentiated health plans, *control* over how much they spend for various health care needs, and *information* to aid their choices."[89]

Herzlinger argues that defined benefit health insurance for employer groups, commonly used today, is structurally flawed because "it causes rapid inflating costs; inadequate coverage and treatment for the sick; lack of quality incentives; and unhappy consumers, providers, payers, and insurers."[90] Consumer-driven health care will remedy these problems by providing the two Cs and one I. First, it will give consumers *choices* by offering numerous highly differentiated health insurance policies that offer various benefits, out-of-pocket expense conditions, and lengths of policies. Employees would be required to purchase, at a minimum, a catastrophic policy. Each of these plans would be subsidized by the employer to exactly the same dollar amount that the employee would put in, or would allow employees to contribute their own money on a pretax basis. This way the cost of the plan would be known by the employer and also the employee. Herzlinger describes how this would work:

> For example, if my employer gives me $6,000 which I perceive as mine, to use for health insurance and care, I may opt for a $4,000 policy that insures me against catastrophically expensive events and accrues the remaining $2,000 in my health savings account so that I can purchase the new eyeglasses and insurance policy that offers long-term care and pharmaceutical benefits I want. The incentives guard against my overinsuring, and the requirement for catastrophic coverage guards against my underinsuring.[91]

Moreover, the insurance companies who offer bundles of care for procedures or illnesses should get paid for the entire bundle rather than for each individual item in it, and they should be able to price their bundles at whatever amount they wish.[92]

Second, consumer-driven health care will offer *information* to the consumer. This information must include user ratings and objective data about both the providers of the health care as well as the health plans themselves. This information will guarantee that "Americans can shop for medical care on the basis of information, not rumor."[93] Equally important is the requirement that all enrollees at a given firm receive exactly the same amount of money toward the costs of each health plan and that they are charged the true price of the plan. Often the price of the health insurance plan reflects factors different from the price it costs the firm. For example, a firm may choose to subsidize a more expensive employee plan through an HMO over cheaper alternatives because it believes the care would be better. But the employee assumes the choice was made because it is cheaper than the alternative plans, so he or she has no notion of how much the plan really costs. Herzlinger argues that when the employee does not know the true price, he or she may sign up for more insurance than actually needed, because the extra benefits are perceived of as "free."[94] If employees have to choose their own plans and are given a specific amount of money to do so, they will choose a plan that is most cost effective.

Third, consumer-driven health care will give people *control* over the value they get for their money. Herzlinger advocates that the price of insurance plan bundles be set by the company paying for the bundle, rather than by the insurance company providing the bundle. Herzlinger claims that the practice of allowing insurance companies to set the prices causes severe problems for people who have chronic conditions that require integrated care. But a consumer-driven health care system "will naturally inspire the evolution of integrated teams. Individuals with chronic diseases or disabilities who can freely choose among differentiated health insurance products will likely opt out of an everything-for-everybody system into one that provides the integrated . . . care that they require."[95] Finally, the payment to insurers and companies that provide the health care must be adjusted by the level of illness of the enrollee. Herzlinger argues that this will create incentives for both insurers and providers to offer policies that cover the sick, "such as multiyear policies that provide payment for health-promoting measures and medical programs."[96]

If these recommendations are followed, according to Herzlinger, costs of health coverage will fall, while the quality of care will rise. Why is this so?

Herzlinger claims that consumer-driven health care will result in integrated information records, which will help people to manage their health and insurance. It will encourage the use of the focused-factory approach and allow them to flourish. What Herzlinger calls "personalized" medicine—that is, drugs tailored to the genetic code of the individual and other technologies that allow the monitoring of various bodily functions—will become incorporated into the health care system, thereby improving its productivity.[97]

For the self-employed or not employed at all, Herzlinger suggests that the innovations brought about through consumer-driven health care will "eventually migrate to the individual market and the wealthier uninsured."[98] The poor and uninsured will be covered by government. Herzlinger suggests that in a "consumer-driven democracy," government has three roles in health care: It regulates the industry to prevent fraud and ensure the financial solvency of the insurers; it requires the dissemination of information, such as audited data about insurers and providers; and it subsidizes health insurance those who cannot afford to pay for it themselves.[99]

Herzlinger does not devote much time to issues of the poor. Basically, she sums up her position by stating,

> And even though others might feel that consumer-driven health care will eventually make health care affordable to all, or that insurance is not really needed because charitable providers will care for the poor uninsured, to me these objections border on fantasies. Health insurance will never be as affordable as a bag of potato chips, and why should poor people scrounge for charitable care while the rest of us can choose the care we prefer? In our prosperous land we should subsidize health insurance for those who cannot afford it so they can obtain health care in the same way as the rest of us.[100]

Finally, Herzlinger cites Switzerland's health care system as an example of consumer-driven health care. In "Consumer-Driven Health Care in Switzerland," a 2004 article in the *Journal of the American Medical Association* cowritten with Ramin Parsa-Parsi, Herzlinger assesses the Swiss system for lessons that can help bring about a dominant consumer-driven health care system in the United States. Herzlinger and Parsa-Parsi note that Switzerland is the only developed country with a long-standing consumer-driven health care system. They find that the Swiss system—which allows consumers to purchase health plans that are independently designed and priced with either their own, their employers', or in the case of the poor, the government's money—is overall quite successful. The system exhibits a 30 percent lower per capita health care cost than in the United States while providing universal coverage and a reasonable quality of care.[101]

Still, Switzerland spends a larger percent of its GDP on health care than most other countries. The authors attribute this fact to the particular preferences of Swiss citizens and available resources. Overall, though, they conclude that the Swiss system "achieves universal insurance and high quality of care at significantly lower costs than the employer-based U.S. system and without the constrained resources that can characterize government-controlled systems."[102]

It is clear from her work that Regina Herzlinger truly cares about trying to find a better health care system for the United States. She has devoted years of her life to researching, contemplating, and writing about how this can be done. She passionately believes in her consumer-driven health care plan. Her dedication to, and work in, this area are admirable.

Still, although her plan is far better than Milton Friedman's, it is deficient in several ways. Like Friedman, Herzlinger has an underlying perspective based on extreme individualism and emphasizing individual human freedom. It is implicit in her writing that the freedom to choose and control are paramount to her argument and the top priorities in her consumer-driven plan. In Catholic social thought, choice and control are seen within a very different context: the impact they have on human dignity and the common good, rather than how they can meet individual desires. Freedom to choose and an ability to exert control are also desirable in that they enable individuals to develop fully as human beings.

Certainly, one of the conditions necessary for personal development is basic health care. Whereas Catholic social thought sees basic health care as a right, Herzlinger does not view it as such. Rather, her concern for health care stems more from the recognition that the present system is economically inefficient, full of contradictions, and therefore in need of a revolution.[103] Although she mentions compassion and concern for people, her writing comes across as being more concerned with economics than with people and more worried about individuals' desires than community needs.

Herzlinger's lack of empathy is also evidenced by her preference for the term *consumer* over *patient*. Using *consumer* deflects from the stern reality of health care. People do not choose to be sick. Most would prefer never to have to use the health care system. But by referring to patients as consumers, Herzlinger lumps sick people with other consumers who purchase televisions, toothpaste, and other consumer goods. Clearly, there is a major difference between an individual who requires and must pay for kidney dialysis and another individual who desires and then purchases a plasma television. Nonetheless, the fact that Herzlinger views all consumers the same belittles the devastation and suffering that disease and illness can bring.

Moreover, Catholic social thought teaches that individual choices and control are judged according to how they affect the common good. Herzlinger shows little, if any, sense of concern for a greater societal, or common, good. Her emphasis is on the individual person and that person's ability to choose and control. Due to her individualistic philosophy, she barely acknowledges the social connectedness of these individuals for whom choice and control are so important. Furthermore, she is not a particularly strong advocate of universal health care coverage. Although she argues that consumer-driven health care will have a trickle-down effect and make health care affordable for the unemployed and self-employed, and though she advocates that government subsidize policies for the poor, she is not particularly concerned with distributive justice. In fact, the term *justice* rarely appears in her work. More importantly, there is little evidence to suggest that if consumer-driven health care were developed, it would trickle down to make policies affordable for the self-employed and the unemployed.

At least Herzlinger admits, unlike Friedman, that markets will not be able to make health care affordable to everyone. Thus, it is apparent that she does indeed share concern for the poor and vulnerable in society. Although she does not devote much of her writing to this topic, she does carefully and concisely state that government should subsidize insurance policies for such groups of people. However, her reasoning for this is not particularly reflective of any deep or nuanced sense of their human dignity. As noted earlier, she just states that the "poor should not have to scrounge for charitable care,"[104] which seems relatively devoid of compassion.

Yet, Regina Herzlinger's consumer-driven health care plan is more compatible with Catholic social thought than Milton Friedman's plan promoting the use of MSAs (or HSAs). At least Herzlinger mentions universal health care and supports a limited role for government in subsidizing health plans for those who cannot afford them. With the prominence she gives to the individual as a consumer who needs choice and control, her work is almost devoid of any sense of the nature of disease and illness, the emotional and personal devastation it can bring, and a just health care system that is necessary to help alleviate the tribulations associated with health problems.

Mark Pauly: Responsible National Health Insurance

Mark V. Pauly is a professor of economics, health care systems, business and public policy, and insurance and risk management at the University of Pennsylvania's Wharton School. He is considered one of the nation's top health care economists.

During the 1990s, when talk of a possible universal health care plan for the United States dominated the health care public policy debate, Pauly, along with economists Patricia Danzon and Paul Feldstein and attorney John Hoff, offered a plan to reform the system. Although the plan was presented by all four people, I will refer to it as Pauly's plan because he calls it "my own . . . proposal" himself and it reflects his vision.[105]

Pauly's "Plan for 'Responsible National Health Insurance'" shows he is no fan of big government. Regarding the government-versus-market debate, he once wrote, "Of course, a government staffed by angels could undoubtedly do a better job than markets run by humans,"[106] the implication obviously being that when humans run a government, the result is not very good. Pauly's view is "that excessive government intervention will make matters worse" in the health care arena.[107] Even with his doubts about government, Pauly is willing to advocate its use to ensure universal health care coverage by giving financial assistance to those who need it.

Pauly begins his health care proposal by stating that a health care plan for reform should be judged by whether it "promotes efficiency and appropriate equity."[108] Efficiency entails minimizing the costs of services provided and electing the right mix of health services, relative to other goods and services, that will allow for the maximum excess of benefits over costs, or the maximum value to consumers. Second, an efficient system does not need to have the lowest costs, as "the appropriate objective is the *right* rate of growth in cost," depending on a comparison of cost and value.[109]

Equity in health care is a more nebulous concept for Pauly. He admits that fairness is difficult to define but settles on a definition based on horizontal equity, where there is "equal treatment of persons with equal real incomes."[110] Thus, someone should not be allowed to pay lower taxes because he or she can get insurance through his or her employer. Pauly also supports vertical equity, which he defines as any income redistribution, accomplished through the tax system, that goes from those with more income to those with less income. Pauly's plan supports competitive markets, avoids the use of the public tax system when possible, and acknowledges present budget constraints.

His plan is based on eight underlying assumptions.[111] First, every person should be able to get health care on a "timely and systematic basis." Next, competitive markets should provide health care, with government intervention only when necessary, such as giving financial help for those who need it. Every citizen should be required to obtain a "basic level" of health insurance. Fourth, the individual person, not the employer, should have the responsibility for obtaining his or her health insurance.

The minimum level of insurance should be based on a family's income. This leads to the sixth assumption: Higher deductibles and copayments would be allowed for those who have higher incomes. Along with this, individuals may also purchase more than the minimum amount of insurance for their income level, if desired, but they must pay for it themselves.

Seventh, Pauly acknowledges that "some modest increase in taxes" would most likely be necessary to pay for the coverage and the tax credits. Still, he argues that his plan is fairer than others because it "relies on a visible and equitable source of financing. This contrasts with the hidden and inequitable financing of mandating employment-based coverage or the present unfair and inefficient system under which care for the uninsured and Medicaid beneficiaries is financed in large part by a *de facto* excise tax on hospital charges paid by the privately insured, without regard to ability to pay."[112] Finally, Pauly's plan assumes that a "vigorous, competitive market in insurance and health care delivery is more likely to create an efficient and high-quality health care system than is one controlled by government."[113]

Starting with these assumptions, Pauly's plan has the following characteristics. It would require mandatory coverage by a basic health plan, meaning everyone would be required by law to purchase basic health care coverage, which could be obtained through either an individual or a family plan. A stop-loss feature would exist, so that the maximum amount of out-of-pocket expenses would be determined by one's income.[114] Insurance plans would be required to provide, at the very least, the minimum benefits determined by government. The benefits would include acute and certain preventative care services, which have been proven to be both cost effective and beneficial to the population. A plan must provide emergency care for an enrollee even in a geographic area different from the area of care specified in the plan. Also, the plans could not have higher deductibles, copayments, or out-of-pocket costs than those mandated by law, based on enrollees' incomes. However, the plans can have additional benefits, at a higher cost, for those people who want more coverage, or people can buy supplemental policies that provide, for example, dental and vision coverage, as long as they can pay for the additional benefits with their own money.[115]

Under Pauly's health care proposal government would designate "fallback" plans for people who do not get coverage in the private market. To find the most cost-effective plans, government would take bids from plans, in a particular area of the country, that offer at least the minimum coverage for a particular premium for each rating category. People who fall into a high-risk category could get fallback coverage through an assigned risk pool that is subsidized by government. The fallback insurer has two purposes. Any individual can use the fallback insurer if he or she chooses. Second, some individuals would be automatically enrolled with a fallback insurer when they do not buy insurance as mandated by law. These individuals would have their insurance premiums collected through the tax system.[116]

The inner workings of Pauly's plan would function as follows. For individuals who are employed, the premium payments and the choice as to whether to purchase benefits over the minimum level would be part of employment negotiations. The employer would have several options. He or she could pay a portion of the group premium, with an implied or express reduction of the enrollee's cash wage. If such a reduction occurs, the premium contribution would be taxed as income to the employee. As alternatives, an express check-off from the employee's paycheck could be made, or the employee might pay the group insurer directly. The employer would report the level of coverage as well as the employer contribution, if any, on the employee's W-4 form. Every employee covered by the minimum insurance plan would receive a tax credit, which would be based on that individual's income—again, including any employment-related premiums.[117]

However, if the employer does not provide a health plan that meets the minimum requirements, then an employee would be required to show evidence on the W-4 tax form that he or she has an policy that adequately makes up the difference, and the proper amount would be withheld from his or her taxes. If the employee does not give any evidence of such coverage, an additional amount of money would be withheld from his or her paycheck to pay for an insurance premium for fallback insurance coverage. In families in which there are multiple workers, only one person would need to get insurance coverage for the whole family.[118]

People who are self-employed would be governed by a universal system of tax credits related to their incomes. Presently, self-employed individuals can deduct a percentage of their health insurance premiums from their taxed incomes. This system would be replaced by a system of tax credits. The self-employed would be required to buy coverage, and then they would be allowed to adjust their quarterly tax estimates to reflect their expected tax credit. If they do not buy coverage, fallback insurance would be purchased "for" them, the cost being added to their quarterly tax estimates.[119]

The dependents of unemployed individuals would be covered by a family plan of someone else in the family who was employed. If this is impossible, then they must buy coverage. If they have adequate taxable income themselves, they would receive the benefit of the tax credit reflected on their quarterly tax estimates. If they do not have enough income to have any tax liability, though, they can file and receive the amount of the tax credit that is owed them.[120]

Pauly acknowledges that many people simply cannot afford to pay for insurance premiums even if they could get a full refund covering the premiums at the end of the year. These individuals would have to go to their local welfare agencies and have their income status verified. Pauly notes that these agencies are already set up to verify incomes, so using them would facilitate the quick plan enrollment of the poor. After verifying that an individual has sufficiently low income to qualify for federal subsidization, the welfare agency would issue him or her a voucher that would serve as an advance to pay for the premium of either a private insurance plan or a fallback plan. The welfare agency would then receive the tax credit due to the individual, and if he or she is receiving other government cash assistance, the amount could be taken out of the cash assistance.[121]

Pauly states that his system would replace the current federal Medicaid system, noting that people who qualify for Medicaid would "probably be eligible for a subsidy equal to the full cost of coverage. . . . A distinct advantage of our plan is that it would eliminate the notch disincentive currently faced by Medicaid eligibles who lose their health coverage completely if they earn income sufficient to raise them above the eligibility threshold."[122] Pauly goes on to argue that this same system could be used to replace the federal Medicare system eventually. He would let people already in the Medicare system stay in, but in the future, as other people start nearing the age of Medicare eligibility, they would enter into Pauly's health plan, rather than the Medicare system.[123]

Pauly's plan also attempts to address the problems associated with risk selection. His plan discusses adverse and preferred risk selection. *Adverse selection* takes place "when the policyholder is better able to anticipate expenses than the insurer."[124] Pauly argues that because his proposal requires all individuals to purchase a specific level of insurance coverage, adverse selection cannot occur in the market for the required coverage. Pauly does, however, admit that adverse selection could occur in the markets providing supplemental insurance. He claims, though, that because supplemental insurance is optional, "it is not a matter of social concern."[125]

On the other hand, preferred risk selection might present problems. *Preferred risk selection* occurs when insurers charge higher premiums to people they deem to be at a higher risk for health problems, and lower premiums for people judged to be at a lower risk. In theory, when the prices of premiums vary in this manner, they discourage risk-taking behavior, such as smoking. Nonetheless, many factors that make an individual a high risk, such as genetic diseases and autoimmune disorders, are simply beyond the control of the individuals who have them. Such high-risk individuals may not be able to get insurance coverage at a price that they can afford. According to Pauly "clearly, a national health insurance plan that relies on private insurance markets must address these possible negative effects of competitive markets."[126]

Pauly contends that the ideal way to address risks would be to have both premiums and tax credits rated on the basis of risk factors. In this way insurance companies would charge people at all levels of risk the actual anticipated cost of coverage, while government also adjusts the tax credits according to anticipated costs. To do this, government and the insurer must have the same information. but Pauly admits that this will probably not be the case. So, if government has less information on people when setting tax credits than the insurer has when setting the premiums, for example, high-risk people within the tax credit categories will end up paying more for coverage.

Pauly examines an alternative to help with these cost differences. The community rating method charges all people the same premium, regardless of their risk factors or health status. Pauly argues that community rating has too many problems. It would undermine insurers' incentives for preferred-risk selection because although they would be making money on low-risk people, they would lose money on high-risk people. Consequently, insurers would have an incentive to avoid high-risk individuals. Moreover, Pauly suggests, although community rating may appear to be an equitable method of insuring people, in actuality it is not because community rating causes the subsidization of premiums for high-risk people by low-risk people. The subsidization occurs independently of income status and ability to pay. Hence, he views such a system as "highly inequitable."[127] The problems with community rating could be lessened by applying a rating for only one of multiple specific actuarial categories, which are established through the use of objective criteria, such as a person's age and the existence of certain diseases. The tax credits could also then be adjusted according to specific categories.

Still, Pauly acknowledges that the set of criteria used by insurers may differ from the ones used by government, causing unfairness. He argues that it is difficult to tell how different the categories might be, how much it would cost to reconcile them, or even whether they would present a serious problem at all. The easiest policy, Pauly suggests,

> would be to use the least interventionist option initially—that is, full and free risk rating for insurers—but permit individuals to claim some adjustment of tax credits according to health-related categories such as age, gender, and specified conditions. Requiring guaranteed renewability of coverage at standard class rates for individuals and small groups could be a condition of the required coverage for all basic plans, so that the problem of high premiums or unavailability of coverage for high risks would diminish over time.[128]

For people who might have been rejected for private coverage, Pauly recommends setting up specific high-risk pools, which are to be subsidized and independent from the fallback insurer. These pools would charge premiums below cost, thereby providing subsidies as well as tax credits, so that their customers would pay premiums within their incomes.[129]

Mark Pauly's "Responsible National Health Insurance" plan is much stronger than either Friedman's or Herzlinger's proposals when assessed in light of Catholic social thought. Catholic social thought teaches that people must be able to develop a full range of human capacities and that this cannot be done without basic health care. Although Pauly never uses the term "human dignity," one of the assumptions underlying his plan is that all people should have access to basic health care. Pauly's plan attempts to "guarantee adequate insurance coverage for all."[130] It does not rely on whimsical thoughts that charities will step in to serve all of the health care needs of the poor and unemployed, nor does it rely on the theoretical proposition that in a free market, health care will trickle down to help those who cannot afford premiums.

Thus, the strongest feature of Pauly's plan is that it strives for equity and fairness. His defining fairness in terms of vertical and horizontal equity reflects his underlying concern for distributive justice. Pauly recognizes that a health care system must be equitable, and this requires that it cover all people. Moreover, its cost to individuals must be determined according to income levels, so that the wealthier pay more for their coverage, while the poor are subsidized for theirs.

Pauly's plan also reflects a philosophy of interdependence in that he recognizes that in a society there is a social obligation to provide basic health care for all. Pauly does not give express reasons for this obligation. He merely states that "not having health insurance imposes a risk of delaying medical care; it also may impose costs on others, because we as a society provide care to the uninsured."[131] Though this may not be an endorsement of Catholic social thought's notion of a common good, at least it recognizes that a societal obligation does indeed exist.

Another positive feature of Pauly's plan is that government is given an important, albeit small, role in implementing his proposal. Pauly acknowledges that this is the most efficient way to "make markets work and to provide financial assistance."[132] Pauly's plan, unlike Friedman's and Herzlinger's, tries to solve the complicated problems that arise with adverse and preferred risk selection as well as community rating. Pauly makes a great effort to analyze the strengths and weaknesses of these issues, to find the fairest method for people who are chronically ill or have severe acute disease to obtain and afford continued health insurance coverage.

Even though Pauly's plan was published in 1991, when health care costs were already a major problem, it does not address the extreme rate of rising costs. On the one hand, his plan represents an admirable attempt to provide universal health care coverage through private markets, government subsidies, and tax credits. He goes to great lengths to guarantee that both out-of-pocket and premium costs will not be overly burdensome for people with low incomes. He also tries to ensure that high-risk individuals can obtain affordable coverage.

Still, Pauly never adequately addresses the essential issue of costs. Pauly does use the usual market theorist argument that efficiency and choice are the solutions to cost containment issues. His definition of efficiency is "minimizing cost of whatever set of services is provided. . . . Efficiency thus reflects a set of choices in which the resources used to furnish all goods and services yield maximum value to the consumers."[133] He goes on to state that the key element in determining whether a good or service is worth its rising costs "depends on a comparison of value to cost."[134] Pauly does not explain exactly how this value will be assessed or how his plan will rein in soaring health care costs.

Mark Pauly's heath care proposal contains several features that make it compatible with Catholic social thought. His plan strives for universal coverage, addresses issues of equity in the financing of the plan, attempts to guarantee that even people in high-risk categories are covered by insurance, and allows a small role for government through subsidization of policies. On the other hand, his proposal does not address soaring health care costs, but merely falls back on market advocates' propensity to rely on competition and a glorified notion of the efficiency it will bring to solve cost problems. The plan fails to analyze other issues, such as the possibile use of supply-side controls to curb high costs and the roles expensive technology and a very broad definition of health have in contributing to soaring health care costs.

Alain Enthoven: Managed Competition

Alain Enthoven is the Marriner S. Eccles Professor of Public and Private Management, Emeritus, of the Graduate School of Business of Stanford University. A widely known and respected economist, Enthoven has been very influential in the health care sector. From 1992 to 1998 he served on the board of the prominent Jackson Hole Group, a network of pro-market economists, health care figures, and insurance industry representatives. He has also been a consultant to Kaiser Permanente for many years.

Enthoven strongly believes that what he calls managed competition is the only kind of health care system that will control costs and provide equitable coverage for everyone in the United States. He uses the term *managed competition* because he believes that an unregulated free market will simply not work. "The markets for health insurance and health care," according to Enthoven, "are not naturally competitive like the markets for transportation, financial services, automobiles or jogging shoes."[135] Enthoven argues that if the health insurance industry is not properly managed, health insurers "would be free to pursue profits or survival by using numerous competitive strategies that would destroy efficiency and equity, and the individual consumers would be powerless to counteract."[136]

Enthoven suggests that there are many reasons that "market failures" occur in the health care sector, with the results being inefficiency and inequity. The most important reason for failure is risk selection, the phenomenon that occurs because expected medical costs, or health risks, can be distributed unevenly among various health plans, and it is to the extreme advantage of the insurer to exclude people who are at a high risk for medical problems. Thus, if an insurer has to quote one premium for all the members of a group, and if the insurer has some choice about who is accepted for inclusion in the group, it is profitable for the insurer to exclude individuals who might have high medical costs. Enthoven contends that there are many techniques for selecting risks, "including medical review of applicants for coverage and refusal to accept people with serious health problems, exclusion or limitation of coverage of care for preexisting conditions, refusal to cover individuals with characteristics thought to be associated with elevated risk of costly illnesses, waiting periods, and manipulation of the coverage to induce the good and bad risks to identify themselves by the coverage they choose."[137] The practice of risk selection among competitive insurers causes inequity because the sick are discriminated against "in the form of underservice and pressure to disenroll," and to make more money, insurers can subdivide groups according to risk and charge higher premiums for the high risk, so that "the sick would pay the full expected costs of their care."[138]

Moreover, Enthoven claims, free market competition among health insurers is inefficient. His support for this claim is very complex. Briefly, because the average individual is risk averse, and the insurer is risk neutral, the economically optimum insurance contract would pay all or part of the first dollar of a medical expense incurred by the individual (providing coverage of all costs, as opposed to having a deductible). This would transfer all of the risk to the insurer. If all people had the exact same risks, optimum first-dollar coverage would exist. But since people do not all have the same risks, insurers use deductibles as a means of separating good and bad risks; therefore, no first-dollar economic equilibrium exists. The lack of optimal first-dollar coverage leads to inefficiency because "the fact that risks are diverse and insurers can select risks using deductibles leads to a departure from optimality," making it impossible to "achieve an efficient solution that would be possible if all persons were of equal risks."[139]

To remedy the inefficiency and inequity of competitive insurance markets, Enthoven proposes managed competition for the health care industry. His major proposal for managed competition was published in 1978. He called his proposal the Consumer-Choice Health Plan (CCHP). Since then Enthoven has continued to refine his ideas and promote them vigorously.

In his original CCHP, Enthoven suggests that the health care industry can take one of two avenues, direct economic regulation or managed competition. Direct economic regulation of the health industry would mean planning controls on hospitals and price controls on both hospitals and physician fees. Enthoven strongly opposes direct economic controls. Like the other three market thinkers discussed in this chapter, he is no admirer of government. Enthoven contends that government represents producer, not consumer, interests. Government controls are not only very rigid but also extremely inefficient when "what every dollar is spent on becomes a federal case."[140] Furthermore, Enthoven maintains that government "does a poor job providing services to individuals" and "performs poorly as a cost-effective producer."[141] When it comes to managing money, government is terrible at it because "in the bureaucratic budgeting system, one strengthens one's case far more by doing a poor job with the budget that one has."[142]

As an alternative to what Enthoven views as the failure of direct economic regulation, his CCHP proposes managed competition, which he claims will "achieve comprehensive care of good quality for all, at a cost we can afford."[143] Managed competition uses microeconomic principles to create a health care system. Managed competition is "price competition, but the price it focuses on is the annual premium for comprehensive health care services, not the price for individual services."[144]

Like the other market organization advocates, Enthoven argues that employment-based health insurance is a failure because "for the most part, employers' purchasing policies do not reward economical health care; they punish it."[145] He characterizes employers' purchasing strategy as containing three themes: a partiality toward a single source of health insurance; subsidization of the most expensive insurers by paying for most or all of the insurance premiums of the plan that the employee chooses, regardless of whether the plan chosen is the cheapest or most expensive; and being self-funding.[146]

Unfortunately, Enthoven claims, these purchasing policies result in high costs and inequity. The single-source policy is based on a "one size fits all" mentality, thereby denying choice to those people who would rather have less expensive care if they could retain the money that is saved by doing so. The single-source policy also impedes provider selection—an element that Enthoven suggests is critical to quality and economy in health care. He argues that the lack of provider selection is one of the major reasons employees revolted against HMOs. Most employers offer their employees a choice of carriers and pay for the whole plan or charge their employee a low percentage of the premium regardless of which insurance carrier the employee chooses. This practice fails to give employees any incentive to choose cheaper insurance providers. Enthoven provides the following example as an illustration:

> An employer offers employees a choice between a preferred provider organization (PPO) with a monthly premium of $200 and an effective HMO with a premium of $150, and it pays 80 percent of the premium of the plan of the employee's choice. That means that this employer subsidizes the high-cost versus the low-cost plan, usually FFS versus capitation at the rate of $40 per employee per month. This punishes the economical delivery system and reduces price elasticity of demand. Inelastic demand means a loss of revenue for cutting price—an incentive to raise, not lower, price.[147]

Finally, the practice of self-funding, or self-insurance, is expensive and inefficient. Enthoven explains that employers use self-funding to control their cash flow and as an investment to earn money when interest rates are high. Under the Employee Retirement Income Security Act (ERISA) of 1974, self-funding employers are exempt from expensive state benefit mandates, and they do not pay taxes on insurance premiums. Also, under ERISA employers' legal liability from employee lawsuits is much more limited than that of insurance companies and HMOs.[148] Yet, self-funding is inefficient because most self-funding plans use a fee-for-service method to pay medical claims. The result is increased costs and decreased incentives to improve efficiency.[149]

Enthoven proposes to solve these problems with managed competition that would allow employers to offer employees a wide choice of carriers and health plans, ensure accountability for the cost of premiums, and offer a choice of the type of health delivery system. Managed competition relies on what Enthoven calls sponsors, which are employers, government entities, or purchasing cooperatives that act on behalf of a large group of subscribers to structure and adjust the market to prevent any effort by insurers to avoid price competition. Sponsors are responsible for establishing rules governing equity, selecting participating plans, managing the enrollment process, creating price-elastic demand, and managing risk selection.

The rules of equity a sponsor should establish include the following. The rules must guarantee that all eligible people are covered, or are at least offered coverage at a moderate cost. All eligible people should have subsidized access to the lowest-priced plan that still meets basic levels of coverage. If someone chooses a plan that covers more than basic coverage, that individual must pay the full premium difference with his or her own money. Once an individual is enrolled, the coverage cannot be cancelled, except for nonpayment or other serious noncompliance with reasonable expectations of behavior. A community rating, or a system very similar to it, should be established so that the same premium is paid for the same coverage regardless of the health status of the individual or group. Finally, no exclusions can be placed on people with preexisting conditions.[150]

Sponsors managing the enrollment process are the key to making this plan work. Sponsors serve as the only entry point to all participating health plans. Thus, a subscriber chooses a plan, notifies the sponsor of that choice, and the sponsor notifies the health plan. The enrollee will be able to switch to a different plan on an annual basis. The sponsor acts as a clearinghouse for the money exchanged for premiums.

Sponsors are also responsible for the creation of *price-elastic demand*, which exists "if the seller increases revenue by reducing prices."[151] According to Enthoven, several means can bring about the price-elastic demand. The key one is not allowing the employer's premium contribution to exceed the price of the lowest-priced plan. The sponsor will decide on the employer's contribution after health plans have submitted their quotes.[152] Another way to guarantee price-elastic demand is to standardize the health plan coverage. Standardization makes comparing the costs of different insurers easier; it discourages segmenting the market into groups of subscribers that choose plans according to what each one covers instead of the cost of each plan; and it allows people to switch plans freely (every year), to save money without losing benefits.[153]

A third way that Enthoven suggests sponsors can create price-elastic demand is by having a national board set standards for outcome information on insurance providers. Such information will help a person decide whether his or her current health plan, or another health plan, is adequate for his or her needs. Sponsors should make sure that this information is readily accessible.[154] Sponsors must also arrange the market to offer health care plans at the individual subscriber level, rather than the employment group level. This lets an individual changing his or her plan much easier than if in a group, where he or she would be dependent on the entire group to change the plan.[155] The final major task for sponsors is to manage risk selection. Enthoven states that the goal of sponsor-managed risk selection is "to create powerful incentives for health plans to succeed by improving quality and patient satisfaction, not by selecting good risks and avoiding bad ones."[156] He sets forth the following ground rules for this process. Health plans must take any subscriber who wants to join, no one can be disenrolled, and anyone must be allowed to re-enroll during the open-enrollment period of the chosen plan. Health plan contracts must all cover the same basic services.

Sponsors must make sure to adjust health premiums for risk. Since high health risks are most likely to occur in different numbers among the various health plans, sponsors must assess the members of different health plans according to such characteristics as sex, age, and disability status, and then estimate what medical costs to expect. Then each plan can be assigned a relative risk index. Surcharges would be applied to premiums of plans that get a favorable risk assessment, and subsidies given to those that do not. Enthoven argues that using surcharges and subsidies will compensate for the usual problems associated with risk selection and "take selection out of the competition."[157]

The final two strategies for sponsor-managed risk selection deal with monitoring. Enthoven suggests that sponsors should monitor the levels of voluntary disenrollment within health plans to determine whether certain plans are using risk selection to get rid of high-risk enrollees. He suggests that a brief questionnaire asking people why they switched health plans will reveal whether risk selection was a factor in the switch. Sponsors must also monitor the quality and availability of specialty care. Health plans can discreetly use risk selection by limiting access to specialists. For example, a diabetic who is not given access to an endocrinologist will not join that particular health plan.[158]

Enthoven is a strong believer in universal health care coverage: "Nobody defends the proposition that people without coverage or money to pay should go without necessary medical care or should be allowed to suffer, be disabled, or die for lack of reasonable care."[159] Hence, his health plan provides for universal coverage for all Americans. Universal coverage could be organized and financed in several different ways. One method is through what Enthoven calls health insurance purchasing cooperatives (HIPCs), which would serve as nonprofit sponsor organizations that would choose the participating health plans and administer health benefit contracts.[160] An HICP would also be a collective purchasing agent for all small employers and individuals in a particular geographic area.

An HICP would oversee the local financing in this system of universal health coverage. One way financing could be achieved, according to Enthoven, is by having employers and full-time employees buy coverage jointly. Part-time employees and "nonpoor" employees, such as early retirees, would pay a tax that would subsidize the purchase of health insurance through an HICP. Enthoven also requires that every household purchase coverage through an HICP or pay an equivalent tax to subsidize coverage for low-income people. He also suggests that payroll taxes or more broadly based taxes can be used to pay for the universal coverage.[161]

Of the four health care plans by market proponents analyzed in this chapter, Enthoven's managed-competition plan is the most compatible with Catholic social thought. One element that sets him apart from all of the other thinkers is his express acknowledgment that pure, unregulated market tactics result in inequitable and inefficient health care systems. Hence, his proposal advocates a system based on competition that is regulated, or in his term, managed.

Enthoven is also a strong advocate of universal health care coverage. He expressly states that no person should be "without necessary medical care or should be allowed to suffer, be disabled, or die for lack of reasonable care."[162] He does not give any specific belief system to support his notion that people should not suffer or die from lack of medical care, but his thought encompasses some underlying commitment to the dignity of the person. Although he does not use the term *human dignity*, Enthoven clearly appreciates that all people, including the poor and vulnerable, need access to health care to live lives that are fully human. This view is reflected in his recent statement that he "would welcome universal coverage as long overdue."[163] One of the ways his plan tries to guarantee universal coverage is by addressing the difficult issues surrounding high-risk health care subscribers. It also looks at ways to stop the insurer practice of risk selection, so that people who are chronically ill or at high risk for health problems can purchase and retain health care coverage.

Enthoven acknowledges that people are socially connected and parts of a greater society. This society has several special obligations toward its members, not just in providing health care. In his early essay on managed competition, when addressing the tension between cutting taxes to encourage job growth and funding public programs, Enthoven argued that "society has other pressing needs: helping the poor, rebuilding cities, energy conservation and environmental protection, to mention a few,"[164] acknowledging the existence of a greater social obligation.

Furthermore, Enthoven repeatedly states that the two major problems with the present health care system are high costs and inequity. Rather than viewing inflation and inequity as merely barriers to *individual* health care, he clearly considers them within the context of their impact on the greater community.

Enthoven finds limitations with capitalism, just as Catholic social thought does. He acknowledges that the free market is not the best system for providing affordable and accessible health care: "A free market does not and cannot work in health insurance and health care."[165] Instead, he argues, managed competition "uses market forces within a framework of carefully drawn rules,"[166] using both the federal government and the private sector to administer his proposal. This language is akin to John Paul II's notion of the juridical framework for economic affairs, in which both the state and private sectors have roles in ensuring economic justice.

This is not to say that Enthoven is highly pro-government. In a 1994 essay opposing the Clinton health care proposal, Enthoven was reflecting on his firsthand experience of working for the Pentagon when he said that the "government is incompetent and ineffective."[167] Still, he does see some role for government in his plan, such as being a sponsor. He advocates a public policy that sets a target for a global budget (defined as lowest capitation rate in each HIPC) relative to GDP to help control health care costs. If the budget grows faster than the target, government should develop and implement interventions to reduce health care spending.[168] Also, government should contract with HIPCs to cover the health care programs that are currently publicly sponsored, such as Medicaid, and to provide for insurance for the uninsured and public employees. Government can also change laws so that sponsors can take necessary measures to create price-elastic demand, as discussed earlier.

Enthoven's proposals, however, fall into some of the same market mindset traps as Pauly's plan. Although Enthoven strives for equity and fairness and acknowledges cracks in the armor of the market when used to provide health care, he still limits his investigation to analyzing efficiency, organizational details, and management tactics to solve our nation's health care woes. Enthoven fails to address, or even to recognize, the deeper values embedded in society that contribute to an inequitable system and to soaring health care costs.

Summary: The Market Organization Approach

I have reviewed the health plans of four different market proponents, representing a spectrum from market purist Milton Friedman to universal health care advocate Alain Enthoven. Clearly, Friedman's health plan is the least compatible with Catholic social thought. With his emphasis on individual freedom, lack of any type of vision encompassing the common good, unresponsiveness to the poor and vulnerable of society, and scarce evidence showing that MSAs (now HSAs) would promote human dignity and the common good (by creating an equitable system that would provide universal access to basic health care), Friedman's cure for health care is full of inequities and lacks justice, as the Catholic social tradition would have it.

Although Regina Herzlinger's consumer-driven health care plan is better than Friedman's, it also emphasizes extreme individualism. Her plan lacks any sense of the common good. Although she does express some concern that the poor receive basic health care and proposes that government subsidize a health plan for the poor, she gives little further attention to the problems of the poor and vulnerable. Rather, her emphasis is on the individual person and that person's ability to make choices and exert control. Moreover, she views health care as merely another example of a consumer commodity that should be treated as such; this trivializes illness and disease. Health care is not a simple consumer good, as Herzlinger would have us believe; therefore, it ought not to be treated as such.

The health plans of Mark Pauly and Alain Enthoven are much more compatible with Catholic social thought. Both of these plans have an implicit respect for the human person and the common good, as evidenced by their recognition of the importance of universal health care. Both of these plans, therefore, have proposals to achieve universal health care. They also attempt to solve problems associated with risk selection, so that universal coverage can indeed be achieved. Equity and fairness are strong underlying themes in both proposals. They also acknowledge, albeit reluctantly, a small role for government in helping to guarantee equity and fairness. Although their proposals, particularly Enthoven's, are extremely complex and would involve a major overhaul of our present health care system, they implicitly contain several of the basic principles found in Catholic social thought: a respect for human dignity, a recognition of social interconnectedness, taking into consideration the existence of some type of greater good, a notion of stewardship of limited resources, and concern for the poor and vulnerable of society.

Yet, like Friedman and Herzlinger, Pauly and Enthoven limit their quests by examining only market practices that will produce a health care system with more efficiency, more individual control, more individual choice, and less involvement of government. This approach tries to tweak the inner workings and details of health care systems to meet the demands of an ideology founded on a massive distrust of government and on the values of efficiency, control, and choice. The fact that government is viewed as the enemy tremendously limits the market organization approach's ability to attain universal health care. Proponents of this approach are so critical of any government involvement in the health care system that they refuse to admit that certain government-run health care systems, such as those in Canada and some European countries, may actually provide decent health care for everyone at an affordable price, much less that we could perhaps learn something from these systems.

Moreover, while some degree of efficiency is both necessary and beneficial to a health care system, too much efficiency can produce a rigid, sterile environment that can erode the trust and compassion essential to a healing community. A similar argument can be made regarding individual control and choice. Although many people desire some control and choice over their health care, an emphasis on personal preferences can hinder any attempt to promote the common good over that of the individual. Individual control and choice also hamper efforts to provide an equitable health system, or one that provides basic health care to all, which cannot be sustained on ideals of individual control and choice. The health care system we presently have in the United States, which favors individual control and choice, is too expensive and inequitable.

Pauly's and Enthoven's plans try to bridge the inequities, but their plans are very complex and most likely politically infeasible. More importantly, though, they do not address the deeper philosophical values underlying the health care system in the United States. In fact, this is the problem with the market organization approach generally. It deals only with the details of the organization and management of the health care system. It argues that the best health care system can be attained through the correct use of medical knowledge and technology within the sphere of institutional settings and medical science.

Yet, organizational details are only one facet of health care. There are other facets to health care that the market organization approach fails to address, such as the goals of medicine and the meaning of health, suffering, illness, and death. These fundamental aspects of life and their influence on the distribution of health care are at the heart of the value dimension approach of Daniel

Callahan. His interest is not merely on how to organize and manage health care but on the underlying value premises that drive our distribution of health care. The next chapter examines Callahan's value dimension approach.

Notes

1. Peterson, "Introduction: Health Care," 12.
2. Muller, *Mind and the Market*, 317.
3. Ibid.
4. Hunt and Sherman, *Economics: An Introduction*, 158.
5. Ibid.
6. Ibid., 159.
7. Muller, *Mind and the Market*, 322.
8. Ibid., 380.
9. Yergin and Stanislaw, *Commanding Heights*, 127.
10. Ibid.
11. Ibid., 130.
12. Technically and historically not a Nobel Prize, the Sveriges Riksbank Prize in Economic Sciences in Memory of Alfred Nobel, established in 1968, is awarded by the same academy as—and is of comparable standing to—the five Nobel Prizes, which were established in 1901, as provided for in the will of Nobel.
13. Friedman, *Capitalism and Freedom*, 13.
14. Ibid., 201.
15. Ibid., 15.
16. Ibid.
17. Ibid., 4.
18. Ibid., 15.
19. Ibid., 27–34.
20. Friedman, "Good Ends, Bad Means," 101.
21. Ibid.
22. Ibid., 101–2.
23. Ibid., 102.
24. Ibid.
25. Ibid.
26. Ibid., 103–4.
27. Ibid., 104.
28. Ibid.
29. Ibid., 105.
30. Ibid., 106.

31. Ibid.
32. Friedman, "How to Cure Health Care."
33. Ibid., 3.
34. Ibid., 4.
35. Ibid., 6.
36. Ibid., 7.
37. Ibid.
38. Ibid.
39. Ibid., 10.
40. Ibid.
41. Ibid., 10–11.
42. Ibid., 11.
43. Ibid.
44. Ibid., 18–19.
45. Ibid., 19.
46. Ibid.
47. Ibid., 22.
48. See John XXIII, *Pacem in terris*, nos. 12, 14, 23.
49. Ibid., n. 54.
50. John XXIII, *Mater et magistra*, n. 67.
51. Second Vatican Council, *Gaudium et spes*, n. 26.
52. Lieber, "The Health Savings Plan You Can't Get," D1.
53. Ibid.
54. Ibid.
55. Herzlinger, "More Market, Less Straightjacket."
56. Herzlinger, "Prix-Fixe Rip-Off."
57. Ibid.
58. Ibid.
59. Herzlinger, *Market-Driven Health Care*.
60. Ibid., xvii.
61. Ibid., xiii.
62. Ibid., 3.
63. Ibid., 25.
64. Ibid., 33–36.
65. Ibid., 37.
66. Ibid., 43.
67. Ibid., 47.
68. Ibid., 82.
69. Ibid., 89.
70. Ibid., 95.

71. Ibid., 104.

72. Ibid., 105.

73. Ibid., 116–21.

74. Ibid., 129.

75. Ibid.

76. Ibid.

77. Ibid., 131.

78. Ibid.

79. Ibid., 134.

80. Ibid., 136.

81. Ibid., 137.

82. Ibid., 148.

83. Skinner, "Focused Factory."

84. Herzlinger, *Market-Driven Health Care*, 163.

85. Ibid., 181.

86. Ibid., 179.

87. Ibid., 186.

88. Herzlinger, "Health Care Productivity," 109.

89. Herzlinger, "Fear and Loathing," 12.

90. Herzlinger, "Consumer-Driven Health Insurance," 74.

91. Ibid., 75.

92. Ibid.

93. Ibid., 76.

94. Ibid.

95. Ibid., 77.

96. Ibid.

97. Herzlinger, "Health Care Productivity," 103–11.

98. Herzlinger, "Consumer-Driven Health Insurance," 98.

99. Ibid., 181–82.

100. Herzlinger, "Scare Stories, Opponents," 182.

101. Herzlinger and Parsa-Parsi, "Consumer-Driven Health Care," 1219.

102. Ibid., 1213.

103. Herzlinger, *Market-Driven Health Care*, xiii–xviii.

104. Herzlinger, "Scare Stories, Opponents," 182.

105. Pauly, "Who Was That Straw Man Anyway?" 468.

106. Ibid., 470.

107. Pauly et al., "A Plan," 6.

108. Ibid.

109. Ibid., 6–7.

110. Ibid., 7.

111. Ibid., 8–10.
112. Ibid., 10.
113. Ibid.
114. Ibid.
115. Ibid., 10–11.
116. Ibid., 11.
117. Ibid., 12.
118. Ibid., 12–13.
119. Ibid., 13.
120. Ibid.
121. Ibid.
122. Ibid., 14.
123. Ibid.
124. Ibid.
125. Ibid.
126. Ibid.
127. Ibid., 15.
128. Ibid., 16.
129. Ibid., 17.
130. Ibid.
131. Ibid., 8.
132. Ibid.
133. Ibid., 6.
134. Ibid., 7.
135. Enthoven, *Theory and Practice of Managed Competition*, 87.
136. Ibid.
137. Ibid., 88.
138. Ibid., 89.
139. Ibid., 90.
140. Enthoven, "Consumer-Choice Health Plan (Part One)," 655.
141. Ibid.
142. Ibid., 656.
143. Enthoven, "Consumer-Choice Health Plan (Part Two)," 709.
144. Enthoven, "History and Principles," 29.
145. Enthoven, "Employment-Based Health Insurance," W3-239.
146. Ibid., W3-240.
147. Ibid., W3-242.
148. Ibid., W3-243.
149. Ibid.
150. Enthoven, "History and Principles," 31.

151. Ibid., 32.
152. Ibid.
153. Ibid.
154. Ibid.
155. Ibid., 32–33.
156. Ibid., 33.
157. Ibid., 34.
158. Ibid., 35.
159. Ibid., 41.
160. Ibid., 35–37.
161. Ibid., 42.
162. Ibid., 41.
163. Enthoven, "Market Forces and Efficient Health Care," 27.
164. Enthoven, "Consumer-Choice Health Plan (Part Two)," 651.
165. Enthoven, "History and Principles," 44.
166. Ibid.
167. Enthoven, "Why Not the Clinton Health Plan?" 132.
168. Enthoven, "History and Principles," 43.

The Value Dimension
Approach to Health Care

The value dimension approach focuses on the values underlying the health care issues that deeply influence the human condition. Whereas the market organization approach emphasizes the details involved in the way health care is organized and managed, the value dimension approach actually evaluates how deeper values—such as the meaning of health, illness, suffering, and death—affect the health care system. These deeper values are overlooked in the market organization approach. Yet, the manner in which they are understood has a tremendous influence over how medicine and health care are viewed and managed.

The major proponent of a values approach to health care is Daniel Callahan. After an overview of Callahan's criticism of medicine and the health care system, this chapter will examine his views on how to remedy health care. I will then assess his approach in light of Catholic social thought. The assessment will determine how compatible the value dimension approach is with Catholic social thought, and it will draw out the differences between Callahan and the market organization approach.

Daniel Callahan is often described as "the limits man." He has spent decades promoting what he calls finite medicine, an understanding of medicine that advocates setting limits in health care. In fact, one of his books is titled *Setting Limits.*[1] At one time he was known as a Catholic writer, and from 1961 to 1968 he was the executive editor of *Commonweal*, a Catholic magazine of religion, politics, and culture. He left the Catholic Church when he realized that he no longer had any religious faith. After leaving the staff of *Commonweal* in 1969, he cofounded the Hastings Center with psychiatrist Willard Gaylin. The Hastings Center was the first think tank in the world to bring critical discussions of bioethical issues to the broader public. Callahan served as president of the Hastings Center until 1996. Today he serves as its director of international programs. He also served on the faculty of Harvard Medical School for several years and is now associated with Yale University.

Over the past twenty years, Callahan has written hundreds of pages on what he calls a finite model of medicine, which is based on an understanding that disease, aging, and death are now, will, and should remain part of the human condition. He argues that a finite model of medicine would be more affordable and sustainable than our present health care system, which is based on an infinite model of medicine, with open-ended goals and no defined end point. Our system now wages an unrelenting war against illness and death, with a great reluctance to set any boundaries on medical hopes and dreams. A finite model of medicine, on the other hand, raises questions about the value and nature of medical progress. It understands that health is not necessarily the highest human value.

Daniel Callahan's Critique of the Health Care System

Callahan argues that the only way to attain sustainable, affordable health care in the United States is by restructuring the goals of medicine and reinterpreting medical progress. He defines an "affordable" system as one "that most people will be able to access," and a "sustainable" one as being "financially viable over the long run (as distinguished from ad hoc coping in a management fashion with financial pressures)."[2] Callahan contends that today's health care system's overly broad understanding of health, along with its view of death as both a biological and moral evil, threatens its equity and economic sustainability. These views of health and death contribute to sustaining a system with infinite desires, which are nurtured by continuous medical progress and new technologies generated by a research imperative. Together these forces are the major source of soaring health care costs and a peril to any equitable distribution of health care.

An Overly Broad Definition of Health

Although Callahan acknowledges that there is no single source of our present health care woes, he argues that the World Health Organization's (WHO) definition of health contributed to the health care mire because it is open-ended. In 1947 WHO officially endorsed this definition: "Health is a state of complete physical, mental, and social well-being and not merely the absence of disease or infirmity."[3] Callahan suggests that by describing health in such an expansive way, WHO opened the door for the notion that, potentially, medicine has no limits. Callahan claims that the WHO definition basically nullified long-standing ideas about health. For example, by including the concept of "social well-being" in its definition, WHO "turns the enduring problem of happiness and well-being into one more medical problem, to be dealt with by scientific means. . . . Good health is, moreover, not even always a necessary condition of well-being. Illness does not preclude happiness or guarantee misery."[4] Rather, he goes on to argue, health is only one part of life and that "while it is good for human beings to be healthy, medicine is not morality. To be healthy and well is not necessarily to be a whole and full person."[5]

Callahan distinguishes between health as a norm and health as an ideal. When viewed as a norm, health can be analyzed in terms of statistical standards, such as levels of organ functioning. The human self (one's sense of having an integrated consciousness, being aware of a personal identity, and having the capacity to act on willed decisions) also has notions pertaining to ideal health, prompting comparisons to current health and implications for the self's sense of wholeness and well-being. Statistical norms help define for the self some of what is good. Callahan contends that the relationship between health norms and health ideals is so strong that "it is impossible, in fact, to draw any sharp distinction between conceptions of the human good—what benefits the self and its goals—and statistical norms of the body."[6] Callahan does not believe, however, that one's self necessarily declines along with one's health. A person with very bad health may still have a strong, active self. An otherwise healthy person, in contrast, can be so dominated by the pain of a toothache as to be beside himself or herself in distraction. Thus, Callahan concludes that "the self and the body are not, it turns out, quite one and the same."[7]

Callahan suggests that the relationship between health and individual happiness is a complicated one, because an individual does not have to be healthy to be happy, and an individual can be healthy but not happy. Hence, the WHO definition of health—which contains the premise that health and human well-being (even "social well-being") go hand in hand—is too broad and simply wrong. Moreover, Callahan argues, the WHO notion of individual well-being "also adds a burden to our thinking about health policy that is bound to increase demands for health beyond prudent boundaries."[8]

Individual needs is a concept that is wide-ranging, and difficult to define precisely in a pluralistic society. Callahan describes three types of needs: merely to exist, or to live; to think and to feel; to act. Within the context of health care, bodily needs correspond to the need to live; without functioning organs we cannot live at all. Psychological needs correspond with the need to think and to feel; without them we are diminished as human beings. The need to act are served by all those functions that allow people to perceive the world, such as vision and hearing, and to respond to it, such as by walking and talking.

In the realm of health care, the categories of human needs serve two roles: They act as benchmarks for describing the common features of all human lives, and they help make the important distinction between curative medicine and caring medicine. Callahan defines curative medicine as treatment "designed to restore our body and its functioning to a state of normalcy in the face of illness, or to forestall a deterioration of capacity."[9] On the other hand, practicing caring medicine means "providing social, psychological, and palliative support when cure cannot be effected (or afforded, as the case may be)."[10]

Yet, according to Callahan, there is a major problem with these notions of health and individual needs. The vision of WHO rests on a very broad idea of health, which encompasses such conditions as social well-being and presupposes that all such needs must be met for health to exist. To make matters even worse, there is an underlying assumption that society has an obligation to meet these individual health needs in some manner. The problem is "that two broad notions are being put together: a wide-ranging notion of individual health, and no less wide-ranging notion of individual need."[11] The combination blocks any attempt by government to define a common good for its citizens, since defining health per individual need implies that only the individuals themselves can adequately define their own needs. Furthermore, it makes it very difficult to create a health care public policy that can define minimal levels of curative medicine, because "the standard of adequacy must not be so low that many individual needs would be excluded, or so high that it would require an unavailable or ridiculously high level of medical advancement and expenditures. Nor can it be a fixed and inflexible standard, good for all times and in all places; it must be relative to the resources and expectations of different societies."[12]

An open-ended understanding of health care combined with endless individual health needs also fuels the idea that people have a right to health care, which Callahan defines as "a legitimate claim of the individual on society to have his or her health needs met."[13] Such a right is very problematic because it is one of many rights claimed in the name of individual welfare. Furthermore, how can we fulfill everyone's health care needs? Callahan argues that within the context of medical progress and its influence on individual medical needs, a right to curative health care is particularly difficult:

> The quest becomes an impossible one, doomed to frustration. The claim that we have a right to healthcare is a claim that our neighbor (ordinarily through the instrumentality of government) has an obligation to provide that assistance necessary to meet our individual health needs. . . . If those needs do not admit, in principle, of any limits or any clear specifications, then there are no boundaries to or claim for healthcare, certainly none intrinsic to the concept of individual need itself. Since we have, moreover, allowed the value of choice and freedom to overshadow other considerations, we have relinquished the possibility of meaningfully distinguishing morally among needs or attaching any fixed priorities to them. The claim of a right to healthcare becomes, therefore, hopelessly vague and open-ended.[14]

Even if a claim to a right to health care were based on a "low" standard of adequacy, such as adequate care or meeting minimal needs, Callahan suggests that these terms still escape definition. He does not propose that we eliminate any and all notions of curative individual needs. Rather, he claims that the concepts of health and medical need must be reevaluated and altered. Any broad notion of curative need, based on meeting the needs of isolated individuals, simply cannot be the focus of health care.

A View of Death as a Biological and Moral Evil

Another major factor contributing to our present health care crisis is medicine's view of death. Callahan says that the line between life and death is growing thinner and thinner. In the past most deaths were caused by infectious disease, accident, or injury and were relatively quick. Between 1600 and 1870, the major causes of death were dysentery, cholera, influenza, plague, smallpox, typhoid fever, and tuberculosis.[15] These illnesses shared one common trait: They were acute, infectious diseases. Either the sick person would die within a relatively short period of time, or he or she would recover without many lingering effects of the disease.

Beginning in 1870, infant and child mortality rates decreased dramatically. With rising life expectancy came another phenomenon: The longer people began to live, the more often they experienced illnesses, and these illnesses lasted a longer time. In Callahan's words, "the price of a longer life has been a sicker life."[16] Now most deaths come as a result of long, chronic illnesses associated with aging. Callahan suggests that this has created a unique situation within the medical profession: It has become difficult to determine when someone is dying. With the slow, chronic nature of most of today's illnesses, the imminence of death is hard to determine.

To make matters worse, the availability of life-extending therapies and technologies make it even more difficult to locate "the gate between life and death."[17] The vanishing line between life and death, as Callahan refers to it, creates havoc within the medical profession. If there is a treatment that will save the life of severely ill patients with a particular disease, but the treatment has only a 5 to 10 percent chance of working, how does a physician decide whether to try it on a particular patient? Callahan argues that because the treatment *might* work, it becomes necessary to treat *all* patients as if they may be among the minority who will benefit from it.

Moreover, today a person could have severe dementia but retain some cognition, or be in a persistent vegetative state and have no consciousness whatsoever. The body can be maintained, however, by using antibiotics to control infections and medically assisted nutrition and hydration to sustain metabolism.

In essence, then, technological advances have changed "the nature of illness to increase the degree and duration of sickness once contracted, to render near-invisible the line between extending a life and extending a death, and then—as a final touch—to render invisible the borderline between a living person and a biologically functioning body."[18] Callahan concludes that the changes in the nature of illness manifest themselves in three specific ways: longer lives and worse health; longer illnesses and slower deaths; and longer aging and increased dementia.[19]

Not only have these changes in the nature of illness made it difficult to determine when a person is dying, but it has become very difficult to know when a person is actually dead. In the past, medicine looked at the cessation of the heart and the lungs as a determiner of death. Now it has added absence of brain activity. Callahan points out that even this criterion for death is not easy to satisfy.

Moral and legal questions surrounding the determination of death abound. When is a treatment "futile"? How can we determine what is medical futility? Is futility determined by the odds that a specific treatment will work? Or do we want to keep the patient's and the patient's family's hopes alive? The challenge in caring for the dying remains to have a "tame death," a concept Callahan takes from French historian Philippe Ariès. A tame death is tolerable, certain, and acceptable.[20]

Along with blurring the line between life and death, Callahan contends medicine has also taken on death as the ultimate enemy, an enemy that must be defeated. Because medicine has been able to cure and treat so many illnesses over the past several decades, it "came to confuse its power to alter, control, or eliminate disease with its power to banish mortality."[21] Hence, another line is blurred. This time it is the line between "human powers and the powers of nature."[22]

There is little evidence to show that before the eighteenth century, it was a duty of a physician to save life. As medicine became more effective in saving and extending life, this altered the view of death. Up until then a sort of fatalism dominated the thinking about life and death. This vision saw death as a natural event that was not, for the most part, under human control. When medicine began to exert some control over the timing and conditions surrounding death, though, then death itself became an evil that had to be eradicated through medical means. By the middle of the twentieth century, medicine had made great strides in extending life expectancies and treating life-threatening diseases. These victories "over" death gave medicine a new goal: to control death, which became a new *moral* obligation. Callahan calls this "the transformation of death from a biological evil to a moral evil."[23] This transition created tension between what we can do to prevent death to what we *must* do to prevent death. In the end all of the weight of the tension fell on the proactive side to make medicine death's terminator.

As a result of this new role, science became consumed with finding the causes and treatments of a vast array of diseases. The underlying premise for this behavior, Callahan argues, was that "if each and every death is caused by a specific disease or condition, why not go after and eradicate them? Eventually there will be none left."[24] Moreover, this desire to control death has resulted in a denial of nature, only to be replaced by "human art and scientific artifice."[25] To illustrate his point, Callahan considers the following four situations and attitudes.

Physicians are often very reluctant to withdraw life-sustaining measures (ventilators, dialysis, insulin, antibiotics, and so on) from patients with irreversible terminal illnesses, because the physicians view this action—not the underlying condition—as killing their patients. It is a mistake, though, to believe that a patient will die from the action of turning off a respirator, instead of dying from the disease that put him or her on the respirator in the first place.

In a related point, physicians are much more likely to withhold a medical treatment for a terminally ill patient than they are to stop a treatment once it has begun. In the former situation, the physician knows that the underlying disease will cause the patient's death, but in the latter case, the physician thinks that stopping the treatment would be what caused the death.

Many research advocates argue that a failure to allocate money to attempt to find cures for certain diseases is tantamount to committing a moral evil that "will leave the blood of the continuing deaths on the hands of those who deny the money."[26]

Many physicians view a dying patient as a victim of medical technologies whose life-sustaining "abilities" are insufficient, instead of the victim of an underlying pathology. Such a viewpoint denies the existence of an inevitable biological death and, instead, sees death as the result of medical failure.

Callahan argues that the distinguishing feature of the foregoing is a blurring of the lines between human actions and an independent human nature. Although he acknowledges that there have been debates about the moral and legal ramifications of acts of omission and commission for centuries, he contends the whole debate has taken on an entirely new dimension. Once medical intervention could actually prevent a death, it became a moral obligation for medicine to do so. So, if intervention fails to keep the patient alive, then it is seen as the actual *cause* of the death. Callahan claims this represents a major change from the traditional distinction between the physical cause of a death by nature, "the impersonal, independent force of biological processes"; and the moral culpability, or responsibility, by anyone "for their actions, or omissions, in response to those processes."[27]

Callahan argues that this blurring between causality and culpability has become "increasingly muddled, intertwined in a tangled knot whose separate strands can hardly be discovered any longer."[28] The result of such an entanglement is a tendency to attribute everything that occurs to human agency. In such a world every act of omission or of commission is of the utmost consequence. Our actions have become so very important, now with the status that nature once held, so everything is viewed as under our control. Hence, Callahan suggests, physicians whose patients die are likely to find fault with their own medical skills, or with medicine itself for having failed to find cures, rather than to accept the inherent dynamism of the underlying pathologies.[29]

Callahan refers to this pattern of blurring the line between the causality of natural biological processes and the culpability of human actions as "technological monism." Callahan views technological monism as an "ingenious way" of also blaming the victim, as if the death were the result of bad human choices instead of an independent work of nature.[30] Death, therefore, becomes our own fault. "By making humans responsible for everything, and making it irrelevant whether they act by omission or commission, we have created an impossibly heavy burden and unbearable burden. . . . If each individual death is understood as in principle a medical and thus a *human* causal and moral responsibility, then the biological status of death itself is rendered inherently uncertain. It continues to reign, but accidentally and contingently, not necessarily."[31]

The underlying impact on health care of making death a moral evil, according to Callahan, is that although death itself cannot be eliminated, medicine will surely do its best to eliminate at least all diseases that cause death. This of course is essentially equal to trying to eliminate death altogether. Callahan quotes William Haseltine, chairman and chief executive officer of Human Genome Sciences: "Death is a series of preventable diseases."[32] From this perspective the causes of death can be controlled, thereby controlling death itself.

Callahan acknowledges there has been some backlash to such a perspective. During the mid-1970s three major efforts attempted to reform end-of-life care and promote a different outlook toward death. There was a movement to encourage the use of advance directives, instructions from patients regarding the type of care they wish to receive when they are dying. The second reform was the hospice movement, and the third was in improving the way medical students are educated on end-of-life care.

Callahan claims that of the three, hospices have been the most successful, although much of their success has been limited to cancer patients. Still, hospices care for over 500,000 patients per year.[33] The major problem with hospices is that most patients come to them much too late, just days before their deaths. As for advance directives, Callahan suggests that they have a mixed record. Since only about 15 percent of people have such directives, their influence on the overall health care system is quite minimal. Even worse, those that do exist are often simply ignored.[34] Regarding the efforts to educate medical students better, Callahan argues that much of what they learn in a classroom situation about end-of-life care may be at odds with their clinical experiences, in which the use of life-sustaining technologies is promoted.

Although these reform efforts have not been particularly successful, Callahan suggests that the common thread running through each is remedying "medicine's characteristic ambivalence toward death: patients' and physicians' confusion about how best to understand and situate death in human life; an unwillingness to accept the coming of death; and the persistence of the turn to intensified technology in response to uncertainty about death."[35]

Regarding death as a moral evil also affects medicine's view of aging, because it—rather than the infectious diseases of the past—is now seen as "the main biological gateway to death."[36] Hence, aging and death have become invariably linked. With low infant and child mortality rates and an increasing life expectancy, viewing death as a moral evil is inseparable from seeing aging as something that can be medically treated or "cured," preventing, as long as possible, the evil from befalling the patient. Callahan points out that although every human ages, much of what is associated with aging can be, and often is, treated by medicine. So, a decline in hearing, a loss of bone mass, failing eyesight, a decrease in lung function, and an increase in blood pressure—all can be medically treated. Although aging is not a disease, it bears so many characteristics of a disease, medicine attempts to respond to it as such.

Society's response to aging is what Callahan calls the "modernization of aging," that is, "the belief that the physical process of aging should be aggressively resisted, and that the life of the aged ought to be transformed from one of old-fashioned disengagement and preparation for death to a continuing active involvement in life and persistent struggle against decay and demise."[37] Although Callahan is not critical of the entire agenda of people holding this view, he recognizes that there are certain realities of aging that challenge the beliefs of modernized aging, such as the chronic illness that more often than not accompanies aging, the persistent poverty of a large portion of the elderly, and the isolation often experienced by elderly people. In fact, Callahan contends, the typical view of modernized aging lacks one essential ingredient: "a sense of collective meaning and purpose."[38] Without some kind of preparation for and acceptance of death, death itself becomes more painful, because it appears pointless and medically unnecessary.[39] Thus, Callahan concludes, the modernization of aging is in essence a call to banish aging by rejecting the difficult questions about the meaning, significance, and value of old age.[40]

A second response to the linkage of death and aging is an attempt by medical science, through the study of genetics, to extend or maximize life expectancies. Yet, the maximization of life expectancies brings with it a multitude of hard questions. Callahan points out that most people who reach the age of 100 years need significant help with their daily activities, suffer from various chronic conditions, and have some form of dementia. Therefore, there are immense social consequences of any increase in life expectancy. The effects on the federal Medicare system is but one such consequence. Callahan observes that in the near future the baby boomers will begin to retire in large numbers, and the proportion of elderly will move from 13 to 18 percent.[41] This will substantially increase the number of Medicare enrollees and create serious problems in government's ability to sustain Medicare at its present level.

Callahan suggests that even larger problems will emerge from continued extensions of life expectancies. A much larger elderly population could have a major impact on society. The elderly generally have greater health care demands, which may drain resources. The age of retirement may have to be increased because there will not be enough younger taxpayers to support even current levels of retirement benefits (not to mention the greater draw on health care aid). With an increase in the retirement age, perhaps fewer jobs will be available for younger people. Issues concerning the social status of the elderly may arise—all this causing intergenerational conflict. In Callahan's words, "Suffice it to say that a society with a much larger proportion of elderly would be a different kind of society, perhaps good, perhaps bad; much would depend on the strategies employed to cope with all the needed changes and how much time was necessary to put them in place."[42]

The Infinity Model of Medical Progress

Another major factor contributing to our health care crisis is what Callahan refers to as the infinity model of medical progress. One of the major forces driving health care costs and inequities is technological innovations, and Callahan says the "research imperative" is the source of these innovations. He claims this is a subject that few in the health care industry want to confront. Nevertheless, Callahan states that the research imperative (and the technological applications that come out of it) "could, for all its benefits, become the source of ever worsening cost pressures and eventually pose a threat to the equitable distribution of health care."[43]

Callahan characterizes the research imperative as

the felt drive to use research to gain various forms of knowledge for its own sake, or as a motive to achieve a worthy practical end. As with technology, where an attractive innovation generates an interest in finding an even better version, research has a similar force. Research generates not only new knowledge but new leads for even more future knowledge; and that is a major part of its excitement. Research has its own internal imperative, that of learning still more, and more.

The research imperative has a continuum of uses and interpretations, each of which I have drawn from many years of reading about research, from listening to its advocates talk about it, and from observing its uses in the public arena:

+ the drive to gain scientific knowledge for its own sake (to understand the human genome)
+ a felt moral obligation to relieve pain and suffering (to find a cure for cancer)
+ a rationale for pursuing research goals that are of doubtful human value or potentially harmful (as some would argue, research to achieve human cloning)
+ a public relations tool to justify the chase after profit (the pharmaceutical industry's defense of high drug prices)
+ the pursuit of worthy goals even at the risk of compromising important moral and social values (hazardous research on competent human beings without their informed consent).[44]

Not until the writings of Francis Bacon and René Descartes in the sixteenth century, according to Callahan, did we have an ideal of medical progress. The idea that death could be defeated by scientific medicine came from Bacon, whereas Descartes predicted that eventually all disease could be overcome.[45] Later Benjamin Franklin, reflecting a similar Enlightenment faith in medicine, wrote, "It is impossible to imagine the height to which may be carried, in a thousand years, the power of man over matter. . . . All diseases may be prevented or cured, not excepting even that of old age, and our lives lengthened at pleasure even beyond the antediluvian standard."[46] Still, it wasn't until the end of the nineteenth century that the ideal of medical progress really gained momentum. Medical research became more systematized through application of the scientific method. A large number of scientific laboratories emerged. German universities and laboratories became the models for scientific research. With the invention of vaccines and several cures for disease in the early twentieth century, a medical research agenda was firmly in place. By the middle of the century, having eradicated many infectious diseases, medicine launched a war against chronic and degenerative diseases.[47]

The underlying theme of all the medical conquests is the same: "The idea of unlimited scientific medical progress, and this idea persists through the present, never weakening in strength but continuing to grow in power. It is an idea that might best be construed as an unlimited vision of knowledge still to be gained and technological application still to be achieved."[48] Callahan suggests the most important ingredient in the research imperative is the success of the medical enterprise itself. He acknowledges that medical science has greatly reduced mortality rates, improved people's health, and helped to relieve much pain and suffering. In other words, medical research works.

So, what is the problem? If it works, isn't it a good thing? Not according to Callahan, who argues that the very success of medical research gives it two paradoxical features. The more health improves and mortality and disability decrease, the greater the drive for more research. So, no amount of success is ever enough. The other paradox associated with the research imperative is the rapid escalation of health standards. The healthier we are, the healthier we want to become. In fact, our standards of personal health continue to rise and rise with no end in sight. So, no amount of physical health and longevity might ever be enough, and such increasingly unbounded expectations would actually be emotionally or psychologically bad for us. Callahan quotes Dr. Arthur Barsky of Harvard, who has observed, "Our medical efforts have by some perverse trick of fate left us with diminished, rather than enhanced, feelings of well-being . . . the healthier we become, the more concerned with health we become. . . . Because our dream is so alluring and our ambitions are set so high, our efforts inevitably leave us feeling disenchanted."[49] Callahan suggests we are caught in a cycle where "the better off we become, the worse we feel; and the worse we feel the more we demand of research; and the more research gives us, the more we ask of it; and when we get what we want we ask for more still."[50]

Not only do we have insatiable appetites for better and better health, but medical research has come to be viewed as a moral obligation, and this is an essential element in driving the research imperative. Callahan argues that, historically, the relief of pain and suffering has always been thought of as an honorable and worthwhile goal of medicine. He acknowledges that the same could be said about medical research when it attempts to help achieve that goal. Hence, research is a societal good.

Yet, what Callahan wants to know is "how high and demanding a good it is. Is it a moral imperative?"[51] To answer that question, Callahan examines the moral principle of beneficence. Philosophically, it has been generally held that there are perfect and imperfect obligations. One's *perfect obligations* are due to the corresponding rights of another. One is obliged to do or provide something for someone else as a result of a contractual agreement or because one's actions or social role generates obligations fulfilling rights that can be claimed against him or her. *Imperfect obligations* are nonspecific. In other words, no person can make a claim that we owe any special duty to carry out some specific action on his or her behalf.[52]

Callahan says that medical research has historically fallen into the category of imperfect obligations. Beneficence requires that we try to relieve medical suffering of others as well as pursue medical knowledge to try to accomplish that task. Yet, it is not a perfect, specific obligation, because no one can claim a right to require that someone else support research that might cure him or her of a disease sometime in the future. Moreover, there is no right held by someone who may get sick in the future to require that research be done to help him or her avoid getting sick.[53] Naturally, Callahan acknowledges the existence of *role obligations*, whereby a medical researcher has an obligation to carry out his or her work to the best of his or her abilities. Still, these are also imperfect obligations because no one can demand that a particular researcher work on his or her particular disease.

Callahan adds that the research imperative usually takes one of two forms: benign or hazardous. In its benign form, the research imperative follows a pattern wherein scientific researchers propose to pursue a specific line of research and usually have a preferred direction in which they want to take it, although it may not necessarily be the "best" or only path to follow. These researchers and their lay supporters suggest that the research may be valuable but do not indicate that it is morally obligatory. If there are some objections to the research on moral or social grounds, the researchers will try to modify their research to respond to the criticisms. If the results of the research do not appear promising, the researchers will move on to another project.

Callahan cites research on violence and behavioral genetics as examples of the benign type. With the social unrest of the 1960s and 1970s, rates of violence rose. Related research took on two major directions. Two doctors at the University of California, Los Angeles, wanted to establish a center for the study and reduction of violence. Initially, the proposal was met with eagerness. Eventually, though, the idea met opposition because rumors prevailed that psychosurgery would be performed on prisoners and other "undesirables." Although the scientific validity of the research was not in question, the project never got off the ground, because of fear that members of certain minority groups might be harmed.

Another proposal aimed at studying violence met a similar fate. In 1970 research began to determine whether males with an extra Y chromosome (in addition to the normal XY pair) have a predisposition to violence. Several objections to the research emerged, including concerns about stigmatizing male carriers of the extra Y chromosome and about informed consent procedures.[54] The XYY research came to a halt without ever concluding whether a causal relationship between violence and the extra Y chromosome exists.

Beginning in the 1960s, behavioral genetics research has tried to determine whether there is a relationship between certain genetic variations and human behavioral patterns. This research has had lots of difficulties gaining acceptance, for several reasons. The main one is that, though most people think that human behavior is influenced by a combination of genetic and environmental factors, there is no agreement about which has greater weight in specific instances. Also, behavioral genetics becomes particularly controversial when, for example, issues are raised linking violence, race, and IQ, or linking homosexuality and such traits as shyness. Thus, the study of behavioral genetics is felt to have the potential for much misuse of the data and stigmatization of, and discrimination against, the subjects and groups they represent.[55] Although the research continues today, its acceptance has been very gradual. Although research into violence and behavioral genetics has many supporters, the researchers have stayed sensitive to critics' claims of potential misuses of the research. Moreover, the proponents have responded quickly to distortions in the media about their work, as well as to excessive enthusiasm by colleagues.[56] One important common feature of both areas of research, according to Callahan, is that they refuse to label the research as morally obligatory.

In sharp contrast to benign research, Callahan argues we have what he calls a morally hazardous form of the research imperative in which proposed research is labeled morally obligatory. Proponents of this kind of research either implicitly or expressly make it clear to the community that the particular research is the only or the indisputably best way to go. Critics of the research are dismissed as either ignorant or biased. If the research is not successful or is slow to show success, proponents use that fact to argue either that more money is needed so the research can succeed, or that ethical concerns are merely holding up the research and should be ignored.

Callahan gives embryonic stem cell research as an example of morally hazardous research. An ethical obligation to cure disease is inherent in the arguments put forth by proponents of this research. Nobel laureate Joshua

Lederberg actually once said to Callahan that "the blood of those who will die if biomedical research is not pursued will be upon the hands of those who don't do it."[57] Similar words have been used by Irving Weissman, one of the leading stem cell researchers.[58]

Embryonic stem cell research has received much hype. Yet, Callahan argues that claims that over a hundred million people can be saved by this research is "inflated advertising language to be sure, but hard to resist."[59]

Researchers and lay proponents claim that, although adult stem cells may be promising, too, embryonic stem cells are theoretically more promising and therefore must be pursued. Even though there are significant ethical objections to embryonic stem cell research, the major one being that an early embryo on its way to a full human life should not be destroyed, the prospect of finding life-saving cures for many diseases trumps the ethical concerns. According to Callahan,

> The scientific claims grow more extravagant, the moral language rises to the highest register, and the objections to the research are mainly explained away rather than being taken seriously. . . . The National Bio-ethics Advisory Commission held that "research that involves the destruc-tion of embryos . . . is *necessary* to develop cures for life-threatening or severely debilitating diseases and when appropriate protections and over-sight are in place to prevent abuse" (emphasis added). The implications of that sentence are that no other line of research can be fruitful, and that there is no abuse in destroying embryos.[60]

Yet Callahan contends such research is not necessary. He is quick to point out that the NIH is already spending hundreds of millions of dollars promot-ing research to find cures for Parkinson's, Alzheimer's, and other diseases. Short of a society-destroying disease, such as a plague or AIDS, Callahan argues that there is no moral obligation to carry out medical research, anyway. Such research may be valuable and worthy, but it is not the ultimate or only social good. Medical research is just one of many valuable human goods—such as food, jobs, housing, and education—that also support human welfare and benefit from research.[61] This is particularly true in developed countries, where most people already have an overall high general level of health. Nonetheless, in all nations there are other social goods that may legitimately compete with health care.

Medical research costs money—lots of money. Callahan notes that the federal project to map the human genome cost $3 billion.[62] The budget of the National Institutes of Health reached $26.9 billion in 2003, and Callahan points out that in 1999 pharmaceutical research cost $24 billion.[63] He expresses dismay over the success of California's Proposition 71, authorizing the sale of $3 billion in bonds to support stem cell research.[64]

It is not that Callahan is against medical research. It is just that he wants research to contribute "to our common good" and move forward "in the most socially sound way possible."[65] The problem, according to Callahan, is that when money is spent on medical research, it must come from somewhere. Usually, it comes from public funds, but often private funds are used, as well. Money that is spent for research is money not spent on other social goods, so scientific progress is now competing with social progress. When it comes to doling out big bucks, "there are plenty of good spending alternatives available to improve our common life."[66]

Callahan cites California's Proposition 71 to make this point. While supporters of this measure were campaigning for money for embryonic stem cell research, California had another story getting wide media attention: 3.8 million adults in Southern California are illiterate. Callahan argues that

> three billion dollars applied to that problem would have almost certain human and economic benefit. That cannot be said of the still-speculative venture that is embryonic stem-cell research. Medical research does not, a priori, have a greater claim to support than many other ways of spending money for social benefits.[67]

Medical research also promotes the development and diffusion of very expensive medical technologies that threaten the equity and sustainability of health care. In the United States, 40 to 50 percent of health care cost increases can be traced to the impact of technology. Callahan notes that a number of studies have suggested that the aging of a population does not, in and of itself, put as much pressure on costs as many people thought. When that demographic shift is combined with a more intense use of technology with elderly patients, however, then the impact is substantial.[68]

In a lecture given in 2003, Callahan mentioned five new technologies for the treatment of heart disease as examples of how much new technologies cost.[69]

Pharmaceutical giant Johnson & Johnson has invented a new stent, called Cypher, which costs around $3,200. The old stent it replaces costs just $900 to $1,200. Expenditures for the new stents are estimated to be $4.6 billion within a year. Another device is the ventricular assist device (VAD) which is used for patients who are not candidates for heart transplants. It costs about the same as a transplant, $160,000, and the estimated added cost of using it for eligible patients is about $16 billion a year. In 2000 there were approximately 35,000 procedures using another heart device, the implantable cardioverter defibrillator. Indications for its use have been expanded to the point that 400,000 people are thought to be candidates for it—to the cost of $24 billion. Scientists are also working on perfecting the artificial heart. If all eligible patients with chronic heart failure were to receive it when it becomes available, estimates are that costs would be around $11.3 billion per year. Finally, aspirin plus clopidogere therapy, useful for secondary prevention of heart disease, would add an incremental cost of $130,000 per quality-adjusted year of life. Therapy using aspirin alone has an incremental cost of $11,000 per year. Callahan acknowledged that he was providing no cost-benefit calculations. Even if just half of the money spent on the new technologies could result in offset savings, though, it would still be a very large amount of money. Moreover, the more expensive the treatment, the more difficult it is to distribute it fairly.

What, then, is to be done about a health care system with an overly broad definition of health, with a vision of death as a biological and moral evil, and an infinity model of medical progress that drives high medical costs, diverts money from other social goods, and thereby threatens the equity and economic sustainability of our health care system? Through a value dimension approach to medicine, Callahan offers an alternate vision: the finite model.

Callahan's Finite Model of Medicine

The major problem with health care, according to Callahan, is that it is based on infinite aspirations; an open-ended definition of health; a relentless battle against illness, aging, and death; and an ideal of unlimited medical progress, driven by a research imperative in which health is the absolute highest value. In other words, we have a medical system that is very reluctant to set any boundaries to medical hopes and dreams. Callahan proposes the following alternative set of values and goals.

The Meaning of Health and General Health Care Priorities

Callahan acknowledges that health is difficult to define and even more difficult to prioritize. On the one hand, health is value laden and therefore influenced by culture. On the other hand, it can also be very subjective. The way in which people tolerate different ailments varies considerably. Health is difficult to define without using some type of evaluative judgments. Given these concerns, Callahan defines health as

> a person's experience of well-being and an integrity of mind and body, the ability to pursue his or her vital goals, and to function in ordinary social and work contexts. That is its positive side. Health is no less characterized by the absence of significant pain, suffering, and harmful disease. By "disease," the main cause of pain and disability, I mean a physiological or mental malfunction reflecting a deviation from statistically standard norms and likely to bring on illness, pain, disability. My definition, then, encompasses the positive and negative traits of "health." It also is far more limited than the famous 1947 World Health Organization definition of health, which encompassed "complete social well-being." . . . Illness may be defined as the individual's experience of pain, suffering, or disability, while sickness refers to society's perception of a person's capacity to function in the usual social roles.[70]

A mere definition of health is not enough for Callahan. He explores the *meaning* of health because it is essential to understand the place health has in human life and in the life of society overall. He begins by asking, "For what ought we to live?"[71] To Callahan there are two major goals of human life. One to try to comprehend what counts as the human good in general. The other is to attempt to know who we are as individual people and what we want to become for ourselves.[72]

Callahan suggests that we all want, psychologically and socially, to develop our capacities to love, work, think, and feel, and to find our proper places within our communities. We pursue good health to enable us to realize our other goals and purposes in life. Good health, taken merely by itself, is basically a worthless good, but it will "have value if purpose can be generated for the life it is meant to serve, and only then can it take its place as a valued means in achieving that purpose."[73] For Callahan the most important questions deal with human ends, such as why we should want to live, for what purposes we should use our gifts, and what is right and wrong. If we have good health but no answers to those questions, our lives would have no meaning, "the worst kind of death."[74]

Health serves not as an end but as a means to finding answers to the essential questions about the meaning and significance of our lives. Good health does this in a couple ways. People want to avoid pain and suffering, which, when too intense, can make life miserable. Also, according to Callahan, health is a "means to our human good in general, and our personal ends in particular."[75] People want good health so they can pursue and achieve personal life goals.

Furthermore, health needs to be thought of within the context of the whole society. Callahan asks, "What is the proper place of the quest for health in devising a societal way of life?"[76] Callahan is openly critical of any society that allows individuals to define their needs in whatever way they want and then expect medicine to fulfill them. Instead, Callahan argues we must redefine the meaning of health and the relationship between individual and societal health. The highest goal of health care in its curative capacity should be "fostering the common good and collective health of society, not the particularized good of individuals."[77]

This requires an understanding of health as a common societal benefit. Callahan contends that health care spending should not be allowed to absorb the GDP at its present ever-rising rate. Health care must not be allowed to trump other societal needs, such as education, public housing, industrial research, roads and highways, and waste disposal.[78]

To determine how to distribute money between competing social goods, Callahan proposes two general principles to determine when society has a sufficient level of health so that monies can be spent on other societal needs. The first principle: "A society will have a sufficient level of health when an absence of good health does not account for a deficiency in the functioning of its major social institutions, and when the great majority of its citizens are healthy enough to carry out their characteristic social roles in the society."[79]

Callahan provides standards to help interpret the sufficiency test. The health of a population is sufficiently good when a great majority, which he defines as four-fifths or more, can carry out a normal range of social functions and enjoy normal interpersonal relationships.[80] He acknowledges that certain population groups will fall below the general average; through the "political process," these groups must then be identified and attempts made to deal with their health needs.[81] Because many health problems of low-income groups have social and environmental causes, he advocates treating those causes, instead of concentrating on health care, to remedy what are systematic, not health, problems.[82]

There is constantly heavy pressure to spend more money on health care to improve health and to minimize disparities. Callahan's second standard is to determine an appropriate balance between the collective societal desire for good health and other societal needs; public policies must be carefully established to reflect this.[83]

Callahan calls this the principle of "full accounting." It acts as a cross-check with the notion of sufficiency. Full accounting means considering the full range of social needs and determining the *long-term* costs of health care. Callahan argues that most health care planning takes into account only short-term costs, such as the cost of a particular type of research to cure a particular disease. A full accounting would consider not only the cost of the research but also the costs of the therapy discovered to treat the targeted disease, its clinical introduction, and its successful implementation. Then the long-terms costs can be calculated. Also, there will always be another fatal disease to take the place of a disease that has been cured. Included in the accounting would be the cost of the other diseases that will eventually kill the people who are cured of the researched disease under consideration. In addition to these costs, related economic and social costs must be taken into account, such as home health care costs for those cured of the disease but who still require long-term additional care.[84]

After considering health among the full range of human and social needs, Callahan's next step is to address the subject of health priorities. Prioritizing caring over curing is closely tied to his definition of health, which includes the belief that the "pain and suffering of individuals should . . . always receive a high priority in the healthcare system."[85] He defines pain as a "distressing, hurtful sensation in the body," while suffering, in the case of an illness, is "a sense of anguish, vulnerability, loss of control, and threat to the integrity of the self." He acknowledges that some pain and suffering can be tolerated, but the relief of all pain and suffering would not be a suitable goal for the health care system. Yet, he contends that it is the vulnerability of illness that most calls for a response from others. He calls this response "one of caring."[86]

For Callahan caring is not a vague or ambivalent feeling. Moreover, it is not a response of surrender because there is nothing else anyone can do for the patient. Instead, caring is an affirmation of a commitment to the well-being of others, a willingness to identify with them in their pain and suffering, and a desire to try to alleviate their situations.[87] A response of caring can involve our personal attitudes, such as patience, concern, and sympathy. Another caring response is the way institutional support is organized to provide comfort, support, and security for the patient in a structured manner.[88] "Caring," argues Callahan, "should always take priority over curing for the most obvious reasons: There is never any certainty that our illnesses can be cured or our death averted. Eventually they will, and must, triumph. . . . Our need for support, for caring, in the face of them is always permanent."[89]

A response of caring, first and foremost, requires an ability to acknowledge our own mortality and shared vulnerability. It requires, therefore, institutions, social structures, and a society that recognizes that all people cannot be cured. Some people will die of their disease and some will be disabled. For example, for the dying a response of caring may require institutional hospice and an in-home program to help patients and their families cope with death. For the mentally ill or mentally diminished, full-time institutional care, in-home care, or counseling may be required, depending on the severity of the incapacity. Callahan acknowledges it is not inexpensive. Still, caring is a finite response to illness and death because it is more limited, easier to implement in social programs, and does not share the infinite goals of medicine to cure all illnesses and forestall death. More importantly, "caring is the foundation stone of respect for human dignity and worth upon which everything else should be built. . . . It is in caring that we can address the uniqueness of persons. . . . When all else fails, as it eventually must in the lives of all of us, a society that gives a priority to caring in its response to individuals is worthy of praise."[90]

The Meaning of Aging, Suffering, and Death

In his book *Setting Limits: Medical Goals in an Aging Society*, Callahan asks, "What kind of sense can be made of old age, of the fact that our bodies change and decline, sicken and decay, and then die?"[91] With medicine's attempt to deny the existence of limits on the human person, Callahan suggests that not only can value be found in the acknowledgement of limits, but such an acknowledgement is necessary to understand the course and trajectory of life and the process of aging. To give meaning to old age, Callahan argues that continuity must be established between the past and the future.

Before explaining how this can be done, Callahan defines *meaning* as "the interior perception, backed by some specifiable traditions, beliefs, concepts or ideas, that one's life is purposive and coherent in its way of relating the inner self and the outer world."[92] *Significance* is "the social attribution of value to old age, that it has a sturdy and cherished place in the structure of society and politics, and provides a coherence among the generations that is understood to be important if not indispensable."[93]

To bring meaning and significance to the aging process, Callahan retrieves the late Calvinist tradition, dominant in America from the end of the eighteenth century to the beginning of the twentieth century. This tradition viewed old age as the end of an important journey marked by vigilance and patience. Old age was a time not only to prepare for death but also to serve one's family and community in preparing for death. Although Callahan acknowledges that we cannot necessarily return to an earlier time, we can reinterpret our definition of a whole life to include the following conditions: Life consists of relatively fixed stages; death may actually be an absolute limit on life; old age is unavoidably marked by decline, so any viewpoint that sees old age as burdensome and marginal must be rejected; and our society would be better off if it shared some common notion of "the whole life."[94]

Callahan suggests several sources of meaning and significance for people who are aging.[95] Linking the past, present, and future gives aging a purpose. The elderly can find meaning in their responsibility to help the young. They are in the best position to integrate the past with the present. Callahan argues that only the elderly can adequately provide coherence to what has happened in the past and what is happening now. The elderly bring experiences that can and should be shared with younger people. Also, the elderly are in the unique position of truly appreciating the present, because their futures are limited. Hence, they are not trying to prepare themselves to be something different from what they are right now. They must make the most of today. This is an art that should be learned and cultivated by people of all ages. Finally, the elderly have an obligation to the future.

Callahan finds this aspect of aging to be the most overlooked. Young people spend most of their time preparing for their future roles. Adults have their own children to raise, and they are responsible to manage the society in which they live. The elderly's most important role is to act as "the moral conservators of that which has been and the most active proponents of that which will be after they are no longer here."[96] Those in their old age are most adept at this role because they alone know what it is like to go from the past through the present to the future.

If there can be meaning and significance in aging, can there also be such in suffering? "No moral impulse," Callahan writes, "seems more deeply embedded than the need to relieve human suffering."[97] The desire to relieve human suffering lies at the heart of compassion and empathy. Callahan's bigger question, however, is whether there is a moral duty to relieve suffering. He suggests one commonly given answer to this question is that we have an obligation if we can do so without a high cost to ourselves and if the suffering is unnecessary.

Yet, what is a "high cost"? Callahan distinguishes between two types of burdens. The first demands that we act to relieve the suffering somehow. This could mean spending time with someone who is ill or spending money on their care. Such demands can be difficult and onerous.

A much more subtle type of burden entails knowing when to accept the suffering as something that cannot or should not be overcome. Callahan argues that honoring moral demands, such as taking an unpopular position on an issue or keeping certain promises, often involves unavoidable suffering. This is the suffering that one must endure out of moral integrity. Moral demands should not be avoided simply because they may inflict suffering. Similarly, no one else has the duty to relieve that suffering—only to help the person bear it. We cannot make it our highest moral duty to relieve suffering. Rather, our duty is "to enhance the good and the welfare of one another. The relief of suffering will ordinarily be an important way to accomplish that, but not always. What we need to know is whether the suffering exists because without it some other human good cannot be accomplished; and that is exactly the case with the suffering caused by living out one's moral duties or ideals for a life."[98]

Callahan distinguishes between psychological and philosophical levels of suffering. The psychological uncertainties of suffering include the fear, dread, and anguish that the sick person has in dealing with an illness and its effect on the his or her life and personhood.[99] Another level of suffering involves basic philosophical and theological questions that have an impact on the meaning of life itself. Here the sufferer asks how the suffering relates to the purpose of human existence, especially his or her own existence.[100]

Callahan argues that physicians should do all that is possible to relieve psychological suffering through palliative care, counseling, and cooperation with the patient's family and friends. But when it comes to the deeper level of suffering, medicine should have no role, "because it has no competence to manage the meaning of life and death—the deepest and oldest human questions—but only some of the physical and psychological manifestations of those problems."[101] It is not responsible to "relieve all the problems of human mortality, . . . to give us control over our human destiny, or to help us devise a life to our private specifications . . . that of complete control over death and its circumstances."[102]

If medicine's job is partly to help relieve psychological suffering, what can we do about the often more profound level of existential suffering? Callahan suggests that suffering related to the search for meaning must be framed in such a manner as to make it bearable. For example, it can be viewed within the whole context of a life that is treasured apart from the suffering, a life full of good memories and rich with relationships built on love and affection. In this way meaning is not in the suffering itself but in the life of which it is a part. That life can be made vulnerable by suffering, but it cannot be destroyed by suffering. Therefore, people can choose to find some rationale for their suffering, which could be in the form of a religious belief or possibly a commitment to respond to pain and suffering with a dignified acceptance of the dependency and fragility that often accompany it.

Finally, how do we find meaning in death? Callahan examines why we fear death in the first place. He suggests the fear is multilayered: the loss of oneself, the loss of relationships, the grief our loss will cause others, and the ultimate *why* in all of it. Why do we have to die? Why must it be this way? A simple biological answer to these questions is that death is necessary for the renewal and continuation of the human species. Yet, tension exists between our status as biological creatures, tied to a cycle that includes birth and death, and our individual self-consciousness, with its will to live.[103]

Still, death is inevitable. Callahan contends that although death may be a generic evil for individual humans, not all human deaths are evil. Death is acceptable under two circumstances. When further efforts to keep the patient alive are likely to distort the process of dying, Callahan writes, "the body has, in that respect, lost its own future."[104] Also, a death ought to be acceptable when "there is a good fit between the biological inevitability of death in general and the particular timing and circumstances of that death in the life of the individual."[105] Callahan defines a premature death as one that comes in youth or well before old age. He defines merciful death as one that comes when the person is no longer able to enjoy the good of life. Furthermore, a death is tragic not only because of terrible surrounding circumstances but also because it has a terrible effect on other people, such as the impact the death of a young child has on the parents.[106]

Callahan acknowledges that his definitions can be problematic. It is difficult to define what is "before old age." If someone dies at the age of sixty-three, for example, is that premature ? To give a more nuanced definition, Callahan describes a premature death as "one that occurs before a person has had a chance to live long enough to experience the main stages of a human life cycle (life, love, work, for instance) and achieve or come close to achieving her or his life projects, or a death that could be averted with no great burden to the individual or society."[107] A death that is neither biologically nor morally wrong should be accepted by medicine as a limit that cannot be overcome, and it should be used as a starting point when analyzing aging and illness.

The Appropriate Goals of Medicine, Medical Research, and Health Care

Not only must the definition of health become narrower and new meaning be given to aging, suffering, and death, but the goals of medicine, medical research, and health care must be redefined to reflect a finite vision. Such a vision will require a rationing of health care to make the system affordable and sustainable. Callahan proposes four major goals of medicine.[108] Although the goals—related to preventative medicine, relief of pain and suffering, distinguishing between cure and care, and death—may appear to be obvious to most people, Callahan argues that they are not so simple. He does not offer any fixed, specific health priorities within each goal, because treatment depends on the stage at which an individual enters the health care system and whether he or she is sick or well and has a chronic or acute condition.

The first major goal should be the prevention of disease and injury and the promotion and maintenance of health. Callahan suggests that because about 50 percent of deaths can be attributed to behavior, such as smoking, prevention should be a major goal of both public health care policy and private medicine. Moreover, medical research should promote greater research in this area. Recently, the Centers for Disease Control and the American Heart Association have begun to spend more of their research budgets on preventative medicine. Callahan argues that the large amounts of money spent on the Human Genome Project should be matched by equally large amounts for behavioral research aimed at preventing disease.[109]

The second goal of medicine should be the relief of pain and suffering caused by maladies. Callahan uses the term "maladies" because disease is not responsible for all pain and suffering. Accidents also cause pain and suffering. The relief of pain and suffering has been one of medicine's goals since its beginnings because pain and suffering are among the most common reasons people seek medical care in the first place.

Medicine should provide care and cure to those with maladies that can be cured, and care to those who cannot be cured. Many diseases cannot be cured but require nonmedical care. Almost everyone will need some type of caring at the end of their lives. Unfortunately, caring has taken a backseat to curing. It is imperative, therefore, that caring medicine receive at least equal weight to curative medicine in all medical settings, including medical research.

The final goal of medicine should be avoiding premature death, yet pursuing peaceful death. Although medicine cannot eradicate death, it can and should attempt to try to reduce the number of premature deaths. More important, though, is the goal of a "peaceful" death, which is not easily defined. The many individual variations have some common threads.[110] A peaceful death is a blend of personal, medical, and social elements. The personal element is the patient's ability to find meaning in his or her own death. The medical element is the practice of palliative care. The social element takes the form of rituals, religious or otherwise, that provide a deeper context for the acceptance of death, such as last rites for the patient and symbols of mourning or services for the family and friends of the deceased. Regardless of how it is defined, according to Callahan, a peaceful death "should not be a goal sought only when nothing more can be done to preserve life or maintain a decent quality of life, when all else fails. It should, instead, be *central to the mission of medicine*, present from the outset of life and not just at its end" [emphasis mine].[111]

A health care system that is affordable and sustainable must use rationing, since everything cannot be available to satisfy everyone's needs and wants for their health care. Callahan has written a great deal on this controversial subject.[112] He advocates a minimal package of health care that would be available to everyone within a fixed system of setting priorities. The minimal package should start with health promotion and disease prevention services, then address emergency and primary care, and move toward the provision of services statistically determined to be the most needed by the average person. Over and above these provisions are other services that would be ranked according to the public's priorities. The public could always allocate more money for health care through an increase in taxes, but if an adequate amount is not allocated, then the public would have to accept further rationing and setting of priorities. Among the most important priorities should be the public's and government's simple refusal to pay excessively high prices for drugs and other health care products and their admonishment against the development of expensive new products. "Industry," urges Callahan, "should receive an unmistakable message that technological developments that make health care increasingly unafford- able are not acceptable."[113]

In summary, Callahan's concept of finite medicine envisions a health care system that would accept a life span that is on average about what it is now, around eighty years, in the healthiest countries in the world. Death would be accepted as an inevitable and necessary part of the human life cycle of renewal. Old age would be accepted as a valuable part of this life cycle. Thus, the primary goal of the health care system should be to help young people grow old, and old people to live out their lives in good physical and mental condition. Further- more, medical research would be understood to function in two primary ways. It would be a way to improve the quality of life within a finite life cycle, while attempting to prevent premature death. Second, research would be only one method among many others, such as improving socioeconomic conditions and the education system, contributing to the health of the overall population.

Catholic Social Thought and Callahan's Finite Medicine

Many elements of Callahan's model of finite medicine are compatible with Catho- lic social thought. Just as Catholic social thought begins with a concept of human dignity, so Callahan relies on a concept of human dignity. Although he mentions respect for human dignity when discussing caring medicine, he does not expressly use the term frequently. Nevertheless, his approach to health care relies on an implicit understanding of human dignity as a vital ingredient. Although Calla- han's notion of human dignity is not based on the Catholic concept of *imago dei*, it does contain a similar understanding of people as having innate moral worth. With his emphasis on finding meaning in aging, suffering, and death, he clearly holds that every person has innate value that must be protected.

Callahan's work reflects a commitment to ensure that all people have access to the basic conditions needed to develop their human capacities. His advocacy of a universal health care system that would guarantee some access to health care for all reveals an anthropology based on respect for the worth of persons. Moreover, Callahan's proposals contain an implicit acknowledgment of humans as socially interdependent beings. He emphasizes finding the proper balance between spending on health care and spending on other social goods, such as education. He also argues for an equitable distribution of social goods, health care being just one good among many others. This position indicates an understanding of the importance of the relationships between individuals and their communities and the political, social, and economic structures that are all necessary for human existence.

A notion of the common good is another essential thread that runs through all of Callahan's work. He vehemently criticizes the rampant individualism that permeates our culture. He views modern individualism, with its emphasis on control and individual needs, as a barrier to universal health care and affordable health care. Callahan urges that medicine establish goals promoting the common good, a good that encompasses the balancing and prioritization of greater social goods while recognizing a limit to individualism and its endless needs and desires. His advocacy of the prioritization of social goods implies an underlying notion of stewardship. Although Callahan does not indicate that social goods, or resources, are gifts from God, he clearly views them as resources that should be distributed justly.

Callahan places a major focus on the poor and vulnerable. As noted, he is a staunch advocate of universal health care. He writes at great length about the most vulnerable people in society: the elderly, the sick, the suffering. The injustices of poverty are important to Callahan, who frequently addresses racial and economic discrepancies in access to health care and in health status.[114] In fact, he finds the high percentage of GDP spent on health care "an insult to the poor (who have no guarantee in the United States, much less in developing countries, of a place at that health-laden table)."[115]

Still, there are elements of Callahan's value dimension approach that vary from Catholic social thought. He objects to regarding health care as a human right because rights come with a connotation of the individualism that Callahan abhors, A right for individuals to have their own specific individual health needs met is impossible, according to Callahan, because such needs are endless. Instead, he claims that if needs are defined in a finite manner, it would then be possible to attempt to meet them.

The notion of health care as a right is problematic even within Catholic social thought. Yet, I do not think Callahan's position is incompatible with

Catholic social thought. Instead, it merely clarifies what the Church actually intends the term *right to health care* to mean. I will discuss this further in the next chapter.

Callahan's finite medicine does not have a Christian framework of meaning per se. He is not a person of faith, so his arguments are based on secular philosophical interpretations and foundations. This does not mean, though, that they are incompatible with Catholic social thought. On the contrary, much of what Callahan argues about the meaning of health, aging, suffering, and death is very compatible with Catholic social thought. However, they can still be enriched with the unique ways of understanding and avenues of meaning found in Catholic social thought.

The final chapter will readdress the market approach to health care and its strengths and weaknesses. Then it will examine Callahan's deeper values, his interpretation of the meaning of health, illness, suffering, and death, and how they affect the health care system within the context of specific Catholic. By examining the strengths of the market and the value dimension approaches from the point of view of Catholic social thought, I will show that a Catholic vision of health care can accept some market mechanisms to curb health care costs but only when used along with certain elements of the value dimension approach.

Notes

1. Callahan, *Setting Limits*.
2. Callahan and Wasunna, *Medicine and the Market*, 269.
3. Callahan, *What Kind of Life?* 34.
4. Ibid., 37.
5. Ibid.
6. Ibid., 39.
7. Ibid.
8. Ibid.
9. Ibid., 43.
10. Ibid.
11. Ibid., 44.
12. Ibid., 45.
13. Ibid., 57.
14. Ibid., 58.
15. Callahan, *Troubled Dream of Life*, 42.

16. Ibid., 43.
17. Ibid., 44.
18. Ibid., 46.
19. Ibid., 47.
20. Ibid.
21. Ibid., 59.
22. Ibid.
23. Ibid., 60.
24. Ibid., 62.
25. Ibid., 63.
26. Ibid., 64.
27. Ibid., 66.
28. Ibid.
29. Ibid., 67.
30. Ibid.
31. Ibid., 68.
32. Callahan, *What Price Better Health?* 67.
33. Ibid., 70.
34. Ibid.
35. Ibid., 70–71.
36. Ibid., 73.
37. Callahan, *Setting Limits*, 26.
38. Ibid., 28.
39. Ibid., 30.
40. Ibid., 31.
41. Callahan, *What Price Better Health?* 81.
42. Ibid., 82.
43. Callahan, "How Much Medical Progress," 885.
44. Callahan, *What Price Better Health?* 3–4.
45. Callahan, "How Much Medical Progress," 886.
46. Callahan, *What Price Better Health?* 12.
47. Callahan, "How Much Medical Progress," 886.
48. Ibid., 887.
49. Callahan, *What Price Better Health?* 33.
50. Ibid.
51. Ibid., 59.
52. Ibid., 60.
53. Ibid.
54. Ibid., 168.
55. Ibid., 169.

56. Ibid., 177.
57. Callahan, "Promises, Promises," 12.
58. Ibid.
59. Ibid., 13.
60. Callahan, *What Price Better Health?* 177.
61. Ibid., 85.
62. Callahan, "Promises, Promises," 13.
63. Callahan, *What Price Better Health?* 31–32.
64. Callahan, "Promises, Promises," 12.
65. Callahan, *What Price Better Health?* 2.
66. Callahan, "Promises, Promises," 14.
67. Ibid.
68. Callahan and Wasunna, *Medicine and the Market,* 250.
69. Callahan, "Medical Technology, Innovation."
70. Callahan, *What Price Better Health?* 87.
71. Callahan, *What Kind of Life?* 106.
72. Ibid.
73. Ibid., 107.
74. Ibid.
75. Ibid., 108.
76. Ibid., 109.
77. Ibid., 110.
78. Ibid., 119.
79. Ibid., 127.
80. Ibid., 129.
81. Ibid., 123.
82. Ibid., 130.
83. Ibid., 131.
84. Ibid., 133–34.
85. Ibid., 143.
86. Ibid.
87. Ibid., 144.
88. Ibid.
89. Ibid.
90. Ibid., 149.
91. Callahan, *Setting Limits,* 31.
92. Ibid., 33.
93. Ibid.
94. Ibid., 40.
95. Ibid., 42–43.

96. Ibid., 43.

97. Callahan, *Troubled Dream of Life*, 94.

98. Ibid., 97.

99. Ibid., 100.

100. Ibid.

101. Ibid., 101.

102. Ibid.

103. Ibid., 164.

104. Ibid., 182.

105. Ibid., 180.

106. Ibid.

107. Callahan, *What Price Better Health?* 91.

108. Ibid., 89.

109. Ibid., 266.

110. Callahan, *Troubled Dream of Life*, 196–97.

111. Ibid., 185.

112. See, for example, Callahan, *Setting Limits* and *False Hopes*.

113. Callahan, "How Much Medical Progress," 890.

114. See for example, Callahan, *What Kind of Life?* 117; *Setting Limits*, 205; and *False Hopes*, 242–43.

115. Callahan, *What Price Better Health?* 276.

A Catholic Vision
of Health Care

The distribution of health care is a long-standing problem in the United States. Costs continue to rise, and the number of uninsured is growing, as well. Although efforts to achieve universal health care coverage have chronically failed, we have yet to reach a consensus on what approach to distributing health care will best address the situation. Market mechanisms continue to prevail as the way to contain costs, and the tradition of Catholic social teaching continues to be critical of the market system for its failures in justice. But as previous chapters have shown, the market organization approach to the funding and distribution of health care is not the only approach, and not everything about the market system has to be condemned.

This final chapter will draw upon Catholic social teaching to show that a Catholic vision of health care can accept some market mechanisms to curb health care costs when they are used along with certain elements of the value dimension approach, as promulgated by Daniel Callahan. This chapter first presents the need for universal access to health care as a requirement of the Catholic social justice tradition. Then it will argue for a Catholic vision of health care that provides universal access by means of some market mechanisms, but only when these are used in conjunction with changes in the underlying values that drive the health care system.

Toward Universal Health Care

The health care system in the United States is in crisis. With an increasingly larger proportion of the GDP going toward health care, double-digit inflation, and a large and ever-growing number of uninsured, the health care system is costing more and more while serving fewer and fewer people. Is this an affront to justice as the Catholic Health Association claims?[1] Does Catholic social teaching support universal access to health care? It does, for respecting the dignity of the person demands it.

People among minority groups are much more likely to be without health insurance than their non-Hispanic white counterparts. African Americans and Native Americans are often uninsured. Approximately 28 percent of African Americans and 36 percent of Native Americans were without any type of health insurance in 2001.[2] Almost one-third of the approximately 44 million uninsured in the United States are Latino.[3] This number is shockingly high, considering that Latinos make up only 13 percent of the total U.S. population. Of all Latinos in the United States, 33 percent have no health insurance.

Although Latinos participate in the workforce at the same rate as non-Hispanic white people, only 43 percent of Latinos are covered by employment-based health insurance, compared to 73 percent of coverage for non-Hispanic white employees.[4] Obviously, one major reason for the disparity is that Latinos often work in professions that do not provide health coverage. For example, they are five times more likely to work in agricultural jobs and are only half as likely to have managerial or administrative jobs.[5] Moreover, they often earn too much money to qualify for federal programs, such as Medicaid. In thirty-five states, even a part-time job that pays only a minimum wage salary can disqualify a single mother from Medicaid.[6] Latinos who are not citizens of the United States face even bigger hurdles when it comes to health care coverage. About 3.5 million Latinos in the United States are not legal residents.[7] Without documentation proving legal status, noncitizen Latinos cannot even qualify for public health care programs.

Minority children are particularly vulnerable to having no insurance. Although such federal programs as Medicaid and the Children's Health Insurance Program provide a much-needed safety net for many children, there are still far too many minority children without any coverage. Of Latino children, 25 percent have no health care coverage at all, while 14 percent of African American children and 7 percent of non-Hispanic white children have none.[8]

There is an even larger question than ethnicity looming when assessing whether access to health care is necessary under the principles of Catholic justice. Statistics show a definite correlation between a lack of health insurance and poor health outcomes. A publication by the Committee on the Consequences of Uninsurance of the Institute of Medicine, *Hidden Costs, Value Lost: Uninsurance in America,* documents the economic and social costs of uninsurance in the United States. The conclusions are quite shocking. Relative mortality rates for insured and uninsured populations, taken from a review of literature on health outcomes, shows a 25 percent greater mortality risk for uninsured individuals between ages one and sixty-five years, compared with those who are insured.[9]

Children without insurance are really hurt. In 2000 approximately 7.6 percent of all newborns were considered to have low birth weight. Newborns covered by health insurance are less likely than newborns without coverage to have low birth weight. Low birth weight is associated with developmental loss. One study of eight thousand children between the ages of six and fifteen showed that children with low birth weight were 50 percent more likely to be enrolled in special education classes.[10] The expansion of health insurance and prenatal counseling has been shown to reduce the rate of low birth weight.[11]

Those older children who do not have health insurance have less access to medical care and therefore do not receive recommended medical and dental care at the same frequency as children with health insurance.[12] Children who are uninsured are at a greater risk than insured children of suffering delays in development that may affect their ability to learn. This in turn affects their earning capacity, as well as their long-term health.

Lack of access to health care and the use of fewer health care services can impede children in many other ways. The most extreme examples are when health insurance provides an avenue to prevent premature death in children. For example, coarctation of the aorta is a fairly common congenital cardiovascular malformation that can be surgically treated or medically managed. This is one of the conditions where a definite correlation can be found between outcomes for the insured and those for the uninsured. One study concluded that infants with a coarctation of the aorta who did not have health insurance were more likely to die, in part because of a failure to diagnose the condition in time to save their lives.[13]

Health insurance coverage is not only a factor in premature death of children but also affects their "ability to achieve normal developmental milestones and to benefit from schooling."[14] The Committee on the Consequences of Uninsurance concluded that a direct connection can be found between the lack of health insurance and a child not fulfilling his or her academic potential. They cite extensive research that shows that several common, treatable childhood ailments—such as ear infections, asthma, iron deficiency anemia, and attention deficit hyperactivity disorder—are often not treated when children have no health coverage. A lack of treatment for these conditions results in illness, school absence, and substandard learning. Asthma is one of the most common chronic illnesses among children in the United States. Approximately 5 million children suffer from this condition, accounting for 3.6 to 11.8 million missed school days each year.[15] Chronic school absence can contribute to poor reading and math skills, frustration, and other factors that play a role in poor academic performance. Not only do such deficits influence a child's ability to achieve academically, but they adversely affect his or her entire economic and health future.

A lack of health care coverage also places a tremendous financial burden on individuals and families. One of the stranger consequences of not having health insurance is that medical charges are usually higher than for those with coverage. The reason is that medical providers, suppliers, and insurers negotiate with each other for prices for various goods and services. This practice often leaves the uninsured, with no bargaining power, paying much higher prices for the same goods and services. An Atlanta attorney, Bryan Vroon, has been trying to get class-action status for a lawsuit challenging the not-for-profit tax-exempt status of a hospital, based on these billing and pricing policies; he described the pricing system in U.S. hospitals as "a Persian rug market of negotiations."[16]

In 2004 a *Wall Street Journal* article covered the plight of one couple facing huge medical care costs. The article describes in detail how a forty-seven-year-old salesman entered the hospital for an emergency cardiac procedure. After a catheterization was performed to unblock arteries, a stent was inserted to increase the blood flow to the heart. The patient had no health insurance. The bills related to his care totaled almost $40,000. A breakdown of the itemized bill showed that the patient was charged exorbitant prices for several of the goods and services. For example, the patient was charged $7,560 for the stent alone. Yet, according to an analyst with a brokerage firm, Cordis, the company that made the stent listed its undiscounted price at $3,195.[17]

The article gave numerous other examples of inflated pricing practices. The sealant used to stop arterial bleeding was billed at $437, when it can usually be purchased for around $200. The gold guide wire, charged at $523, generally costs about $80 to $100. Overall, the entire package of care, including hospital care, medication, devices, and services, was billed at $29,500, but it would have been paid out at $6,000 if the patient had been on Medicaid.[18] One of the main causes for the large size of the bill was that because the patient was uninsured, each of the charges was billed out separately as a line item component of his care, rather than all of the items being billed together as a package, which would have been the case had the patient been insured. Needless to say, the couple has experienced tremendous personal and financial stress as a result of the heart problem.

Financial ruin, often one of the devastating effects of illness, is even more widespread than many originally believed. In 2005 the first extensive study examining the medical concomitants of bankruptcy was published in *Health Affairs*. The results of the study were rather appalling. It found that about half of all bankruptcies filed in the United States were the result of medical expenses that the debtor could not pay. The study concluded that medical problems contributed to bankruptcy for two major reasons.[19] An accumulation of medical bills, including drug costs that cannot be paid, is a big problem, especially considering that almost half of the medical problems found in the study involved chronic illnesses. The other major health care situation contributing to bankruptcy is a loss of income associated with the illness. Some 35.3 percent of bankruptcy debtors were forced to curtail employment because of an illness, often to help care for someone else.[20]

Overall, among families with medical expenses, hospital bills accounted for 42.5 percent of their medical expenses, prescription drugs 21 percent, and physicians' bills 20 percent.[21] Both a lack of insurance as well as gaps in coverage factored as causes of financial problems. Three-fourths of the debtors had insurance coverage at the beginning of their bankrupting illnesses. Yet, a combination of high copayments and deductibles contributed to their financial ruin. One example cited in the study is a debtor who had employment-based insurance. He broke his leg and suffered torn knee ligaments, incurring $13,000 in out-of-pocket costs for copayments, deductibles, and uncovered services, such as physical therapy.[22] Often it is a combination of medical and employment problems that act as major contributors to people's financial woes. The study illustrates with two cases of debtors who had coverage through their employment but lost it. One man had lung surgery and then suffered a heart attack. His hospitalizations were covered by medical insurance, but he was not able to return to his job, which was very physically demanding. He found another job but could not get medical insurance because of his preexisting conditions. Another debtor was a teacher who had a heart attack and missed work for several months, causing her insurance coverage to lapse. Although the hospital wrote off her $20,000 debt, she was still bankrupted because of drug costs and physician bills.[23]

The *Health Affairs* study painted a very dismal portrait of the human face of bankruptcy as a picture of families arriving at the bankruptcy courthouse emotionally and financially exhausted, hoping to stop the collection calls, save their homes, and stabilize their economic circumstances. Many of the debtors detailed ongoing problems with access to care. Some expressed fear that their medical care providers would refuse to continue their care, and a few recounted actual experiences of this kind. Several had used credit cards to charge medical bills they had no hope of paying.[24]

The study concluded that there are four major problems in the financial safety net for people facing illness. First, even short lapses in insurance coverage can cause financial ruin. Second, underinsurance is a serious problem in America. Many families who have insurance were bankrupted by medical expenses that would be considered far below the thresholds of the increasingly popular catastrophic policies, with their high deductibles. Also, for many who have insurance through employment, illnesses often lead to the loss of jobs and subsequent loss of insurance coverage. Finally, because high medical bills and loss of income both contribute to financial ruin, disability insurance and paid sick leave are essential to surviving the financial challenges of illness.[25]

Along with the financial burden of uninsurance comes insecurity, an anxious uncertainty, about the possible consequences of uninsurance. The Committee on the Consequences of Uninsurance labels this uncertainty as "truly a hidden cost of our patchwork approach to health insurance."[26] Health insurance also improves the well-being of individuals and families in other ways often overlooked.[27] Health insurance can provide a much-needed financial security blanket for many families, thereby improving their overall well-being. When a family has health insurance, it reduces the tradeoffs that the family must make between spending money on health care and spending it on other things. Even if everybody in the family is healthy right now, having coverage limits the stress that can accompany the worries and uncertainty about future medical needs and the possible financial devastation if they were uninsured. Low-income families with no insurance have further-restricted financial choices. As income levels fall, families have less and less discretionary income. Hence, the payment for a visit to the doctor represents a larger portion of income and takes a larger share of money away from some other expenditure.

Given the great disparities in health insurance coverage between whites and minorities, the poor health outcomes associated with a lack of coverage, the often ruinous financial consequences of uninsurance, and the stress and uncertainty about the future that a lack of coverage can cause, some type of universal health care system is clearly necessary if we are to protect human dignity and exercise social responsibility for the common good. People cannot develop fully or participate in the economic, social, or political processes that affect their lives without some degree of good health. Moreover, the gospel mandates us to help the poor and vulnerable. The uninsured fall into this category. The poor, with their limited resources, are particularly affected by a lack of access to the health care system. Regardless of income status, people who are injured, ill, suffering, or in pain are very vulnerable. They face the possibility of physical, emotional, and spiritual decline. Such challenges are tough enough to face without also having to bear the financial burden when many doors to medical help are simply closed to them.

Yet, does this mean that in terms of Catholic social thought, a right to health care should exist? Rights language has often been used in a very individualistic way. Charles Curran argues that under an individualistic notion of rights, a right is defined as freedom of action, with the most basic right of the individual being the right to life. In order to sustain life, one can exchange goods and services with others. But a customer has no *right* to someone else's goods and services because their purpose is to sustain the life of the seller or provider.[28]

Another common definition of a right is a legitimate claim of the individual on society to have his or her needs met. Callahan challenges such a definition as too broad and too individualistic, because individual needs can be infinite.[29] Both Curran and Callahan argue that no right to health care exists under those definitions. Still, Curran suggests that a right to health care can be grounded in human dignity:

> Although health care is not the most fundamental need of the human person, it is of great significance. Health is necessary for the proper and full functioning of the life of the person. The right to health obviously means that the individual has the right not to have one's health unjustly attacked by others. In addition there exists within society goods and services of health care, and society is thus faced with the distribution of health care. The right of the individual in distributive justice cannot be considered apart from society and all its goods and members. There are many needs that individuals have—housing, education, health, food, culture, clothing. The basic formulation is simple: a person has the right to that minimum which is necessary for living a decent human life.

The ultimate basis for this right is the dignity of the human person and the fundamental need of the human person. Such a right constitutes a true claim that is obligatory for society to honor.[30]

Nevertheless, if justice requires access to some type of basic health care, do universal systems themselves provide such care? The government-run health care programs of Canada, England, Australia, and New Zealand witness to sufficient ability. A study published in *Health Affairs* in spring 2004 concluded that although the United States spends about twice as much on health care as these countries do, the overall quality of care is no better.[31] These countries provide universal coverage, spend less money on health care than the United States, and have very good health outcomes, but these are primarily government-run health care systems. So, governments can and do manage to run very successful health care systems.

Does Catholic social thought require a purely government-run health care system, or is there room for market practices? Catholic social thought does indeed view government in a positive light. One of the major reasons for this is that, as noted earlier, Catholic social thought considers government an institution for serving the common good. It does not share the market enthusiast's skepticism of government and its ability to provide public services in a positive manner. One major reason for this thinking is that Catholic social thought sees fundamental, intrinsic conflicts between market values and Christian values. As summarized in chapter 3, capitalism is often viewed as treating humans as mere commodities necessary to achieve profit. Moreover, the way that capitalism limits the relationship between the state and its citizens in economic matters allows the state to ignore the needs of the poor while advocating for the wealthy. Capitalism also tends to emphasize the individual's personal needs, rather than acknowledge the individual as living within a web of social relationships and promote the common good. Furthermore, there is little sense of stewardship in a capitalistic economy. Instead of seeing resources as gifts from God to be shared by all, capitalism, with its emphasis on competition and profit, encourages the individual use and control of resources for personal gain. Capitalism thereby encourages consumerism and ignores the plight of the poor and vulnerable in society.

Edmund Pellegrino of Georgetown University, the chairman of the President's Council on Bioethics, argues that market values have no place in health care. He claims that the "healing relationship" cannot exist within the market model of distribution. Contracts, a common feature of market economic systems, "are legalistic, protective agreements between people who do not trust each other. They minimize both trust and commitment. They are not valid when either party is under compulsion to enter the contract, as is the patient who is by the nature of being ill vulnerable, anxious, dependent, and exploitable."[32] Pellegrino goes on to state that market-based models cannot serve a Christian healing relationship, because "healing within the Christian context is inconsistent with the profit-driven care."[33]

The institution of medicine combined with the market tactics used in the United States is oriented toward profit and the maximization of choice and efficiency. Still, are profit, choice, and efficiency necessarily contrary to the values espoused in Catholic social thought, or can they be compatible? German ethicist Ludger Honnefelder argues that the efficient allocation of resources by the market may be an important asset to a health care system.[34] He is right on target. Herein lies the heart of the problem: If a right to health care exists, such a health care system must be both affordable and sustainable. (Here I am borrowing Callahan's definitions of "affordable" as accessible and sustainable, as financially viable in continuing to function and provide necessary health care goods and services.) Hence, the system must be affordable, for the sake of equity. It must be sustainable, because if not, then the system becomes totally ineffective and cannot provide its services to anyone.

One of the biggest problems facing the universal health care systems in other countries is the constant rise in costs. For example, Canada, with one of the most acclaimed universal health care systems in the world, has its cost containment problems. In the 1990s federal and provincial deficits, complaints about mismanagement, and a rising percentage of GDP devoted to health expenditures resulted in large health care budget cuts. By the late 1990s, stability returned to the system, but there are still many problems with it. Number one among them is waiting lists and waiting times. Federal and provincial reports were commissioned to look into the health care system. Overall, these reports reflected a general distaste for market tactics.

Costs are also a continuing problem. Janice Mackinnon, a former finance minister in the Saskatchewan government, said that "health care costs are increasing at a faster rate than the revenue of any government, and other critical priorities are being underfunded in the scramble to cover those costs."[35] Many of the government-run universal health care systems in Europe are also experiencing rapidly rising costs. For example, Sweden and Italy have had to increase the use of copayments to help pay for health care.[36]

Even if we acknowledge the cost containment problem, can Catholic social thought, with its view that government is potentially one of the best entities at promoting the common good, accept a lesser role for government in providing health care? Although the principle of socialization acknowledges that due to the complexities of our modern world, it may be necessary for the state to assume a major role in order to see that human dignity is protected and the common good is promoted, this must be balanced with the principle of subsidiarity, which asks that people look first to smaller, more-local social units to meet societal obligations. Only after seeking assistance at the local level are people encouraged to look for help from larger social agencies or institutions, such as the state or federal government. Proper balance must be forged between a reliance on small social units and government to meet the political, economic, and social obligations required of justice. In his book on Catholic social thought, Kenneth Himes has a nice way of expressing this principle: "No bigger than necessary, no smaller than appropriate."[37]

Here is the tension. If Catholic social thought views government policy as one of the best means of protecting human dignity and promoting the common good, requires some type of universal basic access to health care, and calls for a balance between large national institutions and more localized ones to guarantee this access, is there still a role for private enterprise to play, as in the form of the market? Yes, if government is used to regulate the market and ensure that universal coverage exists.

There are two reasons for this. In terms of just practicality, the United States has a history of love for market ideology and individualism. Given this, along with the fact that efforts to enact a government-run universal health care system (with the exception of the federal Medicare program for the elderly) have totally failed, we are unlikely to see government-run health care. The bottom line is this: In the United States, universal, government-run health care is a political hot potato and has little chance of happening in the near future, if ever. Because Catholic social thought is concerned with justice, requiring universal coverage, and the only way to get such coverage in the United States is through a combination of government oversight and market mechanisms, then it must be considered whether the combination is necessarily the best way to organize the health care system.

Second, certain market mechanisms in providing health care can be compatible with Catholic social thought, but under two major conditions. The mechanisms must meet the minimum standards of justice in contributing to universal coverage and having some type of government oversight. Second, the cost containment issue requires a reevaluation through applying the value dimension approach within a Christian context.

Revisiting the Market Approach

How can market mechanisms meet the standards of justice? In chapter 3 I determined that of the theorists along a spectrum of market approaches to health care, Mark Pauly and Alain Enthoven were the most compatible with Catholic social thought. Now I shall examine these proposals again to determine whether they can adequately provide a universal, affordable, and sustainable system.

In brief, Pauly's plan, with its tax credits and subsidies, strives for universal coverage. Every citizen would be required to obtain a "basic" level of health insurance, based on a family's income, with higher deductibles and copayments allowed for those who have higher incomes. People who fall into a high-risk category could get fallback coverage through an assigned risk pool subsidized by government. Thus, Pauly's plan addresses issues of equity in the financing of the plan, attempts to guarantee that even individuals in high-risk categories are covered by insurance, and allows a small role for government through subsidization of policies.

Enthoven's plan also has universal coverage as one of its primary goals. Sponsors, acting on behalf of subscribers, structure and adjust the market to prevent any effort by insurers to avoid price competition; establish rules governing equity; select participating plans; and manage the enrollment process, creating elastic demand and managing risk selection. Health plans must take any subscriber who wants to join. No one can be disenrolled. Moreover, subscribers must be allowed to re-enroll during the open-enrollment period of the plan of their choice. Surcharges and subsidies will compensate for the usual problems associated with risk selection.

Under Enthoven's proposal, government can act as a sponsor to structure and adjust the market to ensure that it remains competitive and equitable. Government would also be responsible for legislation requiring insurance coverage for all and for the establishment of certain subsidies or broad-based taxes to pay for universal coverage. It would also provide insurance for the uninsured and public employees. Finally, government would help control health care costs by monitoring spending and by implementing interventions designed to reduce health care spending.

Thus, both plans have important roles for government as enforcer and guarantor of universal health care. Without government's requiring coverage and providing some type of monitoring, tax credits, and subsidizations for the poor, no universal system would exist under either proposal. Still, Pauly's plan is too market dependent. He assumes that market competition in health care will keep costs at bay. Unlike Enthoven, who advocates that government should monitor health care costs to keep them at some percentage relative to GDP, Pauly has no provision in his plan for the monitoring of costs. He simply relies on the "invisible hand" of the market to do so.

The problem with this ideology is that it does not work. Callahan is correct when he observes that there are many underlying values driving up health care costs, because the engine driving the health care market is individual choice and desire. Pauly's plan does not address the incessant desire for better health care and more high technology, which are driving up costs. His plan does not provide any method for keeping in check the values that continue to impel costs.

Enthoven's plan has been harshly criticized by those who feel it does not guarantee true universality of coverage. Moreover, as Daniel Callahan notes, both Pauly's and Enthoven's plans are far too complicated for the American public or government, "setting targets for various political and business interest groups and the play of clashing ideologies, and full of enough detail to allow academic critics to inflict upon them the ancient Chinese idea of death by a thousand cuts."[38] Although Enthoven's approach at least acknowledges that someone or something must oversee rising health care costs and take some sort of action to keep them in line, he does not say how they are to be kept down. He does not acknowledge the role of underlying values in driving up costs.

Even though the approaches of Pauly and Enthoven have problems with the role of government in health care, we do not have to go so far as to say that Catholic social thought requires that government run the whole health care system. Market mechanisms are valuable as tools to control costs and help finance the system if used in an equitable way. Although Pauly's and Enthoven's proposals attempt to provide universal health care coverage through heavy use of the market, their major problem is a failure to consider the countless values dominating health care today that influence the affordability and sustainability of the system. Soaring health care costs are a major impediment to universal health care. In the United States, as costs have continued to rise, access has decreased. Even if Pauly's or Enthoven's proposal were enacted and everyone was enrolled in a health care plan, how would the health care system achieve solvency if costs continued to rise at the present rate? How would it remain accessible and effective over time? It simply could not.

State and Local Governments

In 2006 another factor was added to the health care equation: State and local governments are developing their own universal health care plans. In April, Massachusetts passed a new plan for universal health care coverage. Lauded by some as a model for the nation and by others as expensive and unworkable, the Massachusetts plan requires all residents to obtain health insurance by July 1, 2007. Though at this writing it is too early for much professional economic literature to have appeared, the extensive media coverage has shown a fair amount of praise, a no lesser amount of skepticism, and some outright hostility to the plan.

The Massachusetts plan requires all employers with more than ten employees to provide health insurance to their employees or pay the state $295 per employee for each year that they do not provide insurance. People who do not get insurance coverage through their employment yet earn more than 300 percent of the federal poverty level must buy coverage, or they will have to pay income tax penalties. Large insurance pools will be organized by the state so that small business owners as well as individuals can afford the premiums. People earning between 100 and 300 percent of the federal poverty level will receive subsidies to help them purchase insurance. Those earning less than the poverty level would not have to pay any premiums or any deductibles. The law also expands the state Medicaid program so that more children and poor adults are covered.[39]

The plan relies heavily on state subsidies to help pay for the program. It is estimated that subsidies for the poor will cost the state about $720 million a year. However, proponents of the new law point out that the state already sets aside large amounts of money to pay for the costs incurred by hospitals and other health providers when the uninsured receive free care at emergency rooms and other places. This money will now be tapped to help pay for the subsidies. Still, one Massachusetts legislator told a *Boston Globe* columnist that the program is akin to a Hail Mary pass in football because "we don't yet know what it's really going to cost us or where we're going to get the money from."[40] Marcia Angell, the former editor-in-chief of the *New England Journal of Medicine*, noting the absence of cost controls in the new law, predicted, "It will become increasingly unaffordable."[41]

Yet, many in the health care industry applaud the plan. Recently, in an opinion piece for the *Boston Globe*, Phillip Johnston, the chairman of Blue Cross/Blue Shield of Massachusetts, and Nancy Turnbull, its president, acknowledged the challenges facing the new law but proudly endorsed it because "it creates fully subsidized coverage for people. . . . It requires individuals with high incomes who have no health insurance to contribute to a system that cares for all of us."[42] They concluded that "with continued strong collaboration and leadership, Massachusetts can be the first state to show the nation that we can achieve health security for all."[43]

Several other states are looking into similar health care plans. Vermont has passed a health care reform law that helps low-income individuals buy comprehensive health insurance. At the time of this writing, Michigan and New York are considering major health care reform legislation.[44] Reforms are not limited to state governments. In June 2006 San Francisco mayor Gavin Newsom unveiled his proposal to offer a health care plan for all city residents. Revenue for his plan would come from taxpayers, voluntary business contributions, and monthly premiums.[45] The plan was approved the next month.

The success of these reforms remains to be seen. However, three important points should be noted. The state health care reform plans use a combination of government, through oversight and some public revenue, and market mechanisms, such as private insurance and deductibles. Second, in Canada provincial initiatives on health care played an important role in changing the federal viewpoint on universal health care. The Canadian universal health care program actually began in the province of Saskatchewan in 1947 and then moved from there to the federal level. Hence, one could argue that similar initiatives by states in the United States could eventually lead to a federal universal health care plan. Finally, regardless of the various details of specific state and local health care reform plans, the fact that states and cities are actually seeking to have universal health care is a significant event in the history of U.S. health care.

As with the plans of Pauly and Enthoven, the state and local plans have no real provisions for cost control. Even if one or more of these plans can provide universal access with the use of certain market mechanisms for funding, they are not sustainable.

My argument is that a health care system could provide universal access with the use of some market mechanisms to help finance the system and still fulfill the requirements of justice, but only when market mechanisms are used in an equitable manner and in conjunction with changes in the underlying values that drive the health care system. My argument requires a reevaluation of the cost containment issue through the use of the value dimension approach within a Christian context.

Pauly and Enthoven address cost and access problems mainly through changes that attempt to make the health care systems more competitive and efficient. They assume these factors will keep costs down. What they both fail to do is conceptualize the cost problem correctly. On the one hand, changes in the way an institution is managed, organized, and structured can certainly help lower expenses and overall consumer costs. Yet, there are other factors driving the heath care system. With a growing and unrestrained demand, an aging population, and the availability of more high technology and pharmaceuticals, mere changes in the way the health care system is managed and organized are not going to hold costs down. The problem of cost must be reconceptualized in light of two main variables: overall system organization and efficiency, and the values underlying health care. Whereas Pauly's and Enthoven's plans focus on efficiency and overall organization, Callahan's approach to medicine also addresses the values underlying health care. A Catholic vision of health care would combine the value dimension and market organization approaches.

The Underlying Values of Health Care

In order to reconceptualize the cost problem, I will begin by addressing the ends and goals of medicine. Catholic social thought, with its standard of justice and Christian framework of meaning, will help redefine underlying values influencing health care.

The Meaning of Life

In Catholic theology God is the creator and center of value. Understanding that the human being is made in God's image informs us about the relationship between God and humankind and the purpose for our existence. Because we are created in the divine image, we cannot be properly understood apart from God. We are created by a loving God who calls us to be in relationship with him. The *Catechism of the Catholic Church* describes this relationship as follows:

> God, infinitely perfect and blessed in himself, in a plan of sheer goodness freely created man to make him share in his own blessed life. For this reason, at every time and in every place, God draws close to man. He calls man to seek him, to know him, to love him with all his strength. He calls together all men, scattered and divided by sin, into the unity of his fam-

ily, the Church. To accomplish this, when the fullness of time has come, God sent his Son as redeemer and Savior. In his Son and through him, he invites men to become, in the Holy Spirit, his adopted children and thus heirs of his blessed life.[46]

Every individual is born with a distinct personality and set of aptitudes. Everyone must do his or her best to realize these unique gifts, develop them, and use them to the fullest extent possible so that we can direct ourselves "toward the destiny intended" for us by God.[47] Because humans are given intelligence and freedom, we are responsible to fulfill this destiny. The achievement of this self-fulfillment is not optional. Rather, it is required of every human being: "Just as the whole of creation is ordained to its Creator, so spiritual beings should of their own accord orient their lives to God."[48]

Physical life itself is not the ultimate value in Catholicism. This is often misunderstood by many people because of its talk of human dignity and the inherent value of life. Richard McCormick suggests that the meaning and value of life can be formulated as follows: "Life is a basic good but not an absolute one. It is *basic* because, as the Congregation for the Doctrine of Faith worded it, it is the 'necessary source and condition of every human activity and of all society.' It is not *absolute* because there are higher goods for which life can be sacrificed."[49] McCormick quotes Pope Pius XXII, who, in an allocution to physicians in 1957, stated, "Life, death, all temporal activities are in fact subordinated to spiritual ends."[50] McCormick suggests that this can be summed up to mean that "the meaning, substance, and consummation of life are found in human *relationships*, and the qualities of justice, respect, concern, compassion, and support that surround them."[51] The fundamental meaning of life in Catholic thought is found in developing oneself through engaging in relationship with God and other people.

The Meaning of Health

Express definitions of health are elusive in Catholic literature. Richard McCormick attempts to define it when examining what he calls "the responsibilities of health." McCormick argues that the term *health* is both too narrow and too broad to convey a person's responsibilities for it.[52] It is often defined according to its relation to disease, yet the term *disease* itself has various connotations. *Disease* originally meant an inflammatory or degenerative process that, if not treated, could result in serious problems or even death. Then *disease* became defined according to statistics, or a deviation from a so-called normative state. As examples, McCormick mentions diseases whose names are distinguished by the prefixes *hypo-* or *hyper-*; when the thyroid functions more actively than the norm, or excessively, this is hyperthyroidism, and blood sugar below the norm is hypoglycemia.

McCormick goes on to point out that a third concept of disease has developed: disease as an inability to meet societal standards. Hence, people have elective surgeries to enlarge breasts, decrease the size of buttocks, and reduce facial wrinkles. McCormick suggests this notion of disease reflects a society that does not accept nonconformity.

Finally, McCormick suggests that all sorts of desires are becoming "medical" problems for which people are increasingly seeking treatment. He mentions the definition of health held by the World Health Organization (WHO): "Health is a state of complete physical, mental, and social well-being and not merely the absence of disease or infirmity."[53] He agrees with Daniel Callahan and argues that the WHO definition is far too broad, and if followed, "the quite preposterous situation could arise where a person's sense of well-being is threatened by the size of his or her car. The appropriate medical judgment would be a prescription for a Chrysler Imperial to replace one's Dodge Dart."[54]

The term *health* can also be too narrow. McCormick argues that a narrow concept of health ignores the whole person. It relies on using high-tech equipment to care for the dying, instead of giving personal care and comfort. It depersonalizes medical treatment, so that a sort of insensitive apathy governs medical decisions, where "'orders not to resuscitate' are too often carried out as if they were orders to do nothing—not even care."[55]

Although he does not offer a specific definition of health, McCormick's critique of what the term conveys can provide us with some ideas of what health is not. Health is not merely the absence of an inflammatory or degenerative process, or the lack of a variation from a statistical norm. It also does not mean meeting the whimsical desires of the individual to have a younger or more attractive physical appearance. Nor does health comprise the *complete* emotional, psychological, physical, and social well-being of an individual; yet, it is more than something that affects solely the physical body, because the emotional, spiritual, and psychological components of the human being cannot be reduced to the merely physical.

Daniel Callahan's definition of health encompasses both the heart of Catholic thought on the meaning of life as well as McCormick's notion of what health means. The first part of Callahan's definition describes health in terms of "a person's experience of well-being and an integrity of mind and body, the ability to pursue his or her vital goals, and to function in ordinary social and work contexts."[56] This part of his definition recognizes, as does Catholic social thought, that humans are multidimensional, have unique gifts to offer the world, and are relational, in that they must be able to operate within various spheres of society.

Callahan's definition goes on to say that health

> is no less characterized by the absence of significant pain, suffering, and harmful disease. By "disease," the main cause of pain and disability, I mean a physiological or mental malfunction reflecting a deviation from statistically standard norms and likely to bring on illness, pain, disability, while sickness refers to society's perception of a person's capacity to function in the usual social roles.[57]

The second part of his definition addresses McCormick's concern that health not be defined too narrowly. Here Callahan makes the important distinction between "disease" and "sickness." Whereas disease is viewed as a deviation from the statistical norm, sickness refers to societal perceptions of an individual's ability to function, to *relate* to others. Callahan is therefore offering a definition of health that acknowledges the entire human person—the depth of his or her being, along with the need to develop capacities and to use them in relation to others and to society.

Within a Catholic vision of health care, the meaning of health would be very different from what it is in our present health care system. Health would be seen as an essential part of human life but not the goal of life, which is to develop capacities in order to fulfill oneself in relationship to God. Some level of good health is required in order to achieve this goal. Hence, health is one of the means to help one attain full personhood. It is just *one* of many such vehicles, not the ultimate human value. It is an important value, but it does not trump all of the others.

This relative value of health implies that other societal goods, such as education, housing, employment, and the arts, should not automatically take a backseat to health care when it comes to funding and research priorities. On the other hand, good health is important enough for our commitment to respect human dignity to require that all people have access to some level of health care. This moral requirement makes universal coverage a social mandate.

A commitment to universal health care would make a minimum standard of coverage available to all. Because it would be impossible to restrict wealthier Americans from buying additional coverage or from paying for services out of pocket, some disparity in access will remain. Nevertheless, at least all Americans will have access to basic care.

Even a commitment to universal coverage would not necessarily halt spending an excessive amount of the GDP on health care, however, nor would it ensure that spending would not be allowed to grow rapidly. In order to achieve an economically sustainable universal health care system, certain market mechanisms could be used, but within limits. For example, some form of rationing of health services, particularly the use of expensive technologies, would have to be devised that set specific priorities. Public health, for instance, would be valued over the desires and needs of the individual. Hence, public health programs, preventative care, and primary care would be major parts of the health care system.

In addition to setting limits on market mechanisms, other changes would have to occur within our social consciousness and practice of medicine. For instance, aging would have to be more accepted as a natural aspect of the life cycle, not considered some disease to be cured or postponed. Along with old age would come certain restrictions on medical care, so that overly aggressive care and an overuse of technologies and pharmaceuticals would not occur. Death and certain types of suffering would have to be accepted over aggressive interventions. The health care profession would have to make some major changes. Medical schools, for example, should offer a broader curriculum that emphasizes preventive care, the care of those with chronic illnesses, and palliative care, so that the commitment to caring would be on par with the commitment to cure. Such changes in our understanding of health would have a significant impact on restricting the demand for expensive technologically supported health care.

The Meaning of Illness and Healing

In an essay on a Roman Catholic perspective on healing, bioethicist Edmund Pellegrino outlines the roots of the Catholic imperative to heal. In the Old Testament, Yahweh is a healer. He heals Miriam of her skin problems and King Hezekiah of a deadly disease. Yahweh also shares this healing power with others. For example, Elijah is able to bring the widow's son back to life and to cure

Naaman of his skin ailment.[58] In the New Testament, a call to heal is rooted in the many episodes in which Jesus heals all sorts of people. One of his most frequent activities, after preaching about salvation, was to heal the sick.[59] Pellegrino shows how Jesus told the Parable of the Good Samaritan to instruct his followers on how to care for others: "Like the Samaritan, they were to care for the sick with solicitude even when they were strangers and even when it meant inconvenience and cost to the Samaritan."[60]

With his emphasis on healing, according to Pellegrino, Jesus altered the ancient world's view of illness as a punishment for sin and a sign of the inferiority of the sufferer. Jesus demonstrated that illness was not disgraceful and that sick people were not to be shunned. Pellegrino quotes Matthew 25:39–40 to make this point: "I was sick and you visited me. Inasmuch as you do this unto one of the least of my brethren, you have done to me." Pellegrino contends that this teaching by Jesus gave the sick individual a "preferential position" and created for the Christian community a duty to care for the sick and the poor. Hence, healing is a vocation, a calling from God to help those who are sick.[61]

Within the Christian perspective, healing is more than merely repairing the physical body. We understand illness as a challenge not only to one's physical security but even to one's emotional and, frequently, spiritual well-being. The sick person asks questions about God and his or her relationship with him, like "Where is God in this?" and "Why is God doing this to me?" Healing entails not only attempts to cure the disease or illness and to relieve pain and suffering, but restoring one's relationship with God.[62]

Pellegrino says that providing hope to those in despair is essential to Christian healing: "For the Christian, healing can occur even as the patient is dying and suffering, right up to the last moments."[63] Because "the sick will always ask Job's question: Why, Lord? Why me? Why now?" Pellegrino suggests that we cannot answer those questions for them, but we can give them comfort and consolation "when it becomes clear, as it did to Job, that God does not owe us an answer."[64] He quotes the late Joseph Cardinal Bernardin of Chicago, who suffered from pancreatic cancer, to describe this aspect of Christian healing:

> Our distinctive vocation in Christian health care is not so much to heal better or more efficiently than anyone else; it is to bring comfort to people by giving them an experience that will strengthen their confidence in life. The ultimate goal of our care is to give to those who are ill through our care a reason to hope.[65]

The goal of hope, according to Pellegrino, is to contradict the despair that occurs when humans are faced with their finitude. There is nothing like a serious illness or impending death to cause an individual to confront his or her limits as a human being. When we are forced to confront our limitations as finite beings, only a God who has promised that we will not face our problems alone can offer us hope.[66]

The challenge for the health care community in living out its vocation as healers is to surround those who suffer with love in order to help absorb the terror of their suffering. In so doing, it assures them in their hopes that they will neither lose their dignity nor be abandoned by the community. Living through suffering with hope can be the way we face the limits of our mortality. By accepting our human condition, we may avoid the application of medical procedures that only prolong the dying of a rapidly deteriorating body, and we may spare excessive expense for our families and the social community.

The Meaning of Suffering

The meanings of illness and healing are not complete without some way of finding meaning in the experience of suffering. For almost all people, especially those who are ill, the experience of suffering needs some sort of explanation, some meaning for its occurrence. Everyone suffers in some form at some point in their lives. The cause, length, and degree of suffering vary with the individual. Still, we *all* suffer. And yet, we ask, Why me? Do I deserve this suffering? What is God's role in it?

The ancient Greeks tried to find meaning in suffering. Who cannot be touched by these profound words of Aeschylus (525–456 BC) in his drama *Agamemnon*: "Drop, drop—in our sleep, upon the heart sorrow falls, memory's pain, and to us, though against our very will, even in our own despite, comes wisdom by the awful grace of God."[67] The quest to discover the meaning of suffering has continued into more recent times. German philosopher Friedrich Nietzsche wrote, "Happiness and pain are inseparable twin brothers: they grow together or remain small together; it is impossible to have one without the other."[68] And then there is the often-quoted story by Dostoevski wherein Ivan Karamazov states that he wants to return his ticket to life back to God because the world is filled with too much innocent suffering. Ivan is repulsed by the notion that suffering has some type of utilitarian value, in that it is justified from the perspective of higher harmony.

Jewish psychiatrist Viktor Frankl, who spent several years in Nazi concentration camps, concluded that we can find meaning in our suffering because to live is to suffer and to survive is to locate meaning in the suffering.[69] He argued that if there is meaning to life, then there must be meaning in suffering. He recommended that people stop dwelling on the meaning of life and instead ask what life expects from us. By concentrating on this and acknowledging that we have free will, a person can endure suffering, because he or she can choose to make it unique opportunity to fulfill his or her destiny: "When a man finds that it is his destiny to suffer, he will have to accept his suffering as his task; his single and unique task. He will have to acknowledge the fact that even in his suffering he is unique and alone in the universe. His unique opportunity lies in the way in which he bears his burden."[70]

As the dialogue on suffering continues, there may seem to be no adequate answers. In his book on suffering, Peter Kreeft argues that with the age of modernity, suffering came to be viewed as a "scandal, a problem to be conquered rather than a mystery to be understood and a moral challenge to be lived."[71] Kreeft suggests that modernity has lost faith in ultimate meanings—the meanings associated with the things humankind did not invent, such as life and our inner beings.[72] He distinguishes between man-made and non-man-made suffering. Because man-made suffering, such as war, is created by humans, it is easier to understand how it occurs. With the non-man-made kind of suffering, though, we have alienation and despair. Because non-man-made suffering is not dependent on humans, Kreeft reasons that no meaning can be found for it without appealing to the supernatural reality, or God. Because modernity denies the existence of God, though, it cannot deal with non-man-made suffering.[73]

The problem of suffering is troublesome even for the Christian believer. In his book on suffering, *A Different God: A Christian View of Suffering*, Kristiaan Depoortere suggests that suffering is such a difficult concept for humans because it "hides" God. The fact of suffering in our lives raises questions about the existence of God. It raises questions about what can be perceived as God's silence in view of suffering. For the Christian who is called by the Gospels to relieve suffering, its existence can create anxiety about how to help the sufferers of the world.[74] Depoortere looks to theologian Dorothee Soelle, to whom suffering descends on humans and causes them to feel alienated, which she characterizes as powerlessness and meaninglessness. Because suffering also causes people to feel isolated, Soelle suggests that only through solidarity, a sharing of the suffering with other people, can suffering be overcome.[75]

Christianity brings a unique outlook on suffering. One of the most famous stories of suffering is the classic Old Testament story of Job. Satan receives permission from God to test Job's faith. In the beginning of the story, Job loses everything he has, including his own children. He is afflicted with sores all over his body. Although he never loses his trust in God, Job does experience a tremendous struggle to accept his tribulations. In chapter 3 he rants about his suffering and curses the day he was born:

> Let the day perish wherein I was born,
> and the night which said,
> 'A man-child is conceived.'
> Let that day be darkness!
> May God above not seek it,
> nor light shine upon it.
> Let the gloom and deep darkness claim it.
> Let clouds dwell upon it;
> let the blackness of the day terrify it.
> (Job 3:3–5)

> Why is light given to him that is in misery,
> and life to the bitter in soul,
> who long for death, but it comes not,
> and dig for it more than for hid treasures;
> who rejoice exceedingly,
> and are glad, when they find the grave?
> (3:20–22)[76]

In chapters 4 through 27, Job tries to discuss his trials with three of his friends, but they repeatedly blame him for his problems. They argue that God is always just, so if Job is suffering, he is being punished for something. Job must somehow be at fault for all these horrible things to happen to him, even if he is not aware of what he did to deserve them. Yet, this is not the God in whom Job has so much faith, and Job refuses to endorse his friends' claims. He does not believe in a retributive God. Although angry and shaken, Job stays true to his faith in a God who is a redeemer:

> For I know that my Redeemer lives,
> and at last he will stand upon the earth;

and after my skin has been thus destroyed,
then from my flesh I shall see God,
whom I shall see on my side,
and my eyes shall behold, and not another.
My heart faints within me!
(Job 19:25–27)

Eventually, God restores, twofold, all that Job had.

Depoortere's interpretation of Job holds that seeing God as a ruler who rewards good behavior and punishes bad behavior has been prevalent for centuries. However, this view is heavily flawed. When one examines the world and the people in it, one sees that there is no clear connection between immoral behavior and divine punishment.[77] We all know of people who behave in immoral ways but who never seem to be punished for it. We also know people who live righteous lives and still have horrible things happen to them. Job is such an example. He was a righteous man who had to endure horrible suffering. Jesus Christ is another example of a victim of injustice.

Depoortere argues that an image of God as a cold judge is unfair to both people and God. It encourages people to be complacent and guilt ridden. It also portrays God in purely moralistic terms, with God seen as a more powerful version of a human father. Yet, Depoortere suggests this is not the God who is revealed in Jesus Christ: "He is different. . . . He is not a God of revenge; He is not a God of bookkeeping retribution."[78]

Still, what kind of being is God? And what is the meaning of suffering? Through the use of the framework of Adolphe Gesché, a theologian who wrote on suffering, Depoortere concludes that God is the enemy of suffering. The Bible is a record of God's struggle against evil. More importantly, "If human beings fight suffering, they are not left alone. God fights on their side (*cum Deo*)."[79] God does not tolerate evil. Rather, God bears it with people. This fact that the individual confronting suffering is not alone is a key concept because evil's strongest power comes from its ability to alienate fellow human beings both from each other and from God.[80]

The birth, life, and death of Jesus Christ give a much richer understanding of human suffering. Depoortere calls the Passion of Christ "the story of God as a fellow-sufferer."[81] Jesus died an ugly death. It was not the obviously valiant death of a war hero or the headline-grabbing passing of an acclaimed celebrity. No, he died a bloody, brutal death, having been abandoned by most of his closest followers. On the Cross, according to Depoortere, we see a God who is near the sufferers. Because God does not save Himself, but rather endures the pain of the Cross, God identifies with the sufferers as a compassionate God. But the story does not end there. In many ways it begins there. The story goes on to tell of a passage through the suffering. It tells a story of victory over the suffering.

According to Christian teaching, suffering, especially during the last days of life, is an opportunity for the Catholic health care community to take a clear stand on the importance of family and community support. Facing the experience of suffering is a time to emphasize the role of interpersonal and spiritual values in defining the meaning of life. It is also the time to place technologically supported end-of-life care within a holistic perspective on life and death, which includes our commitment to solidarity and justice in providing health care to all sectors of society. These values, tied into the way we respond to suffering, are keys to a Catholic vision of health care.

The Meaning of Death

All human beings share at least one thing in common: One day each of us will die. This is a fact of our existence, and each person must deal with it in some way. An awareness of death presents a unique challenge to the person. Catholic thought views death as "the end of earthly life."[82] For those who die in the grace of God, death is the participation in Christ's death and Resurrection.[83] Death is not the end of a person's life; it is the transition to a new life with God, our final end.

Christianity teaches us that Jesus died on Good Friday. Depoortere points out that the Gospels portray a rather dismal picture of disappointment among his disciples on that day. They struggled to accept the reality that their leader was dead. On Sunday the women went to his tomb to annoint his body. Upon their arrival they were shocked to see that the stone in front of the tomb had been moved away and Jesus was not there. Mary, the mother of James, thought that his body had been stolen and hidden. Then a stranger, a man that many do not immediately recognize, began to make appearances. Mary Magdalene was the first to recognize this man to be the risen Lord. Depoortere characterizes the Easter rising of Jesus as a triumph over suffering.[84]

The belief that Christ overcame death through the Resurrection, and that we will too, is foundational to Christianity. It gives us a sense of hope and a new meaning to life and death. For a Christian, death is not the end, nor is it an enemy to be defeated at any cost. It is part of a larger redemptive process.

Depoortere suggests that there are three major ramifications of the Resurrection of Jesus.[85] It reaffirms the powerful relationship based on love between God and humankind. It teaches us that if we continue to live in relationship to God, the divisive effects of suffering and death will have no power over us. Second, the promise of the resurrection of the dead affirms the importance of relationships to other people. What we have done for each other will continue to live on. Third, the Resurrection of Jesus represents the final corrective to suffering and death.

Within this view of death and resurrection, Catholic social thought formulates its criteria for making decisions about prolonging life. The Catholic tradition charts a course between the extremes of physical vitalism's "never say die" attitude and utilitarian pessimism's readiness to end a useless or boring life. Physical vitalism sees physical life as the absolute good and death as an unnatural enemy to be avoided at any cost. Utilitarian pessimism supports taking life that is not useful in ways determined by society. The Catholic tradition affirms life as a basic good, a necessary condition for every other human activity, but not as an absolute good that must be sustained at all cost.

This twofold awareness is enshrined in the "ordinary/extraordinary" means standard dating back to the sixteenth century.[86] Ordinary and extraordinary means of life support distinguish between obligatory and optional treatment. The Catholic tradition recognizes that not all technologies are equally appropriate and useful for prolonging life, and not all means need to be used by those who are sick or dying. The 1980 *Declaration on Euthanasia* admitted that the terms *proportionate* and *disproportionate* may now be preferable to avoid the ambiguities of the traditional formulation of this standard.

The key point of the distinction is that technology or means of treatment alone cannot be classified simply according to type; instead, it must be judged by the circumstances relative to the patient's capacity to benefit from the treatment. A means is disproportionate (extraordinary) whenever it is not medically useful, too burdensome to use, or even too expensive. As the *Declaration on Euthanasia* would have it, any particular means of prolonging life must be evaluated in terms of "the treatment to be used, its degree of complexity or risk, its cost and possibilities of using it, and comparing these elements with the result that can be expected, taking into account the state of the sick person and his or her physical and moral resources."[87] Even a means already in use can be withdrawn if it "carries a risk or is burdensome."[88] Refusing a means of life support in such a case "is not the equivalent of suicide; on the contrary, it should be considered as an acceptance of the human condition, or a wish to avoid the application of a medical procedure disproportionate to the results that can be expected, or a desire not to impose excessive expense on the family or the community."[89]

Even with this distinction as a guide, just how far a patient, or the patient's proxy, must go to prolong life is not easy to determine. Because the key to what is morally required are the circumstances of the individual patient, not the treatment in question, different patients with the same diagnosis and treatment plan can decide differently. There is no "one treatment fits all" approach to determining what must be done to prolong life.

This ambiguity is especially acute when the proposed treatment is medically assisted nutrition and hydration. The 2004 edition of the *Ethical and Religious Directives for Catholic Health Care Services* of the U.S. Bishops stipulates, "There should be a presumption in favor of providing nutrition and hydration to all patients, including patients who require medically assisted nutrition and hydration, as long as this is of sufficient benefit to outweigh the burdens involved to the patient."[90] Over the past several years, different theologians and bishops have offered differing views about whether and when medically assisted nutrition and hydration should be considered disproportionate treatment. The issue is particularly difficult in the case of a person diagnosed as being in a "persistent vegetative state" (PVS), unable to perceive his or her own condition and appreciate the prospects of an extended life. Is extending life in such a condition a benefit or burden to human dignity? Should the interests of others—the family or others who lack access to medical care—be relevant in determining whether a means is disproportionate, especially when the tradition has related the welfare of the patient to family and communal relationships?

These questions about using medically assisted nutrition and hydration in the case of PVS were not clearly resolved by the March 2004 allocution of Pope John Paul II. In his address "Life-Sustaining Treatment and Vegetative State," Pope John Paul II said that providing medically assisted nutrition and hydration for PVS patients is morally obligatory "in principle." Some Catholic ethicists expressed shock at what seemed to represent a "significant departure from the Roman Catholic bioethical tradition with respect to both the method and the basis upon which such decisions are made."[91] But in November 2004 in his "Address of John Paul II to the Participants in the 19th International Conference on the Pontifical Council for Health Pastoral Care," the pope reaffirmed to a Vatican conference on palliative care that decisions about treatment must be based on the benefit/burden assessment enshrined in the traditional standard. Because neither the 1980 Vatican declaration nor the *Ethical and Religious Directives* governing Catholic health care facilities in this country have been revoked by recent Vatican statements, we ought not abandon the proportionate/disproportionate distinction.

Rather, the judicious application of the proportionate/disproportionate-means standard, as it has been interpreted over a long-standing tradition, is a Catholic contribution to how we can respect the dignity of the patient and make joint use of resources. Studies show that dying in America continues to be both expensive and overly burdensome. A publication by Last Acts, a national coalition to improve end-of-life care, found that the high percentage of elderly people who spend a week or more in intensive care units at the ends of their lives suggests that they may have received overaggressive care.[92] Moreover, although physicians believe that 90 to 95 percent of pain can be controlled, at least half of dying patients report being in pain.[93] Hospice programs are underutilized, and palliative care units and physicians trained in palliative care are in short supply. Approximately 75 percent of those over sixty-five years old die in either a hospital or a nursing home, even though a great percentage of Americans say they want to die at home.[94] In 2000 only 42 percent of all hospitals had a formal pain management program, 23 percent had formal hospice programs, and a mere 14 percent had palliative care programs.[95] Truly, we do not deal with death well. We take dying people out of their homes, away from the public view, only to have them die in strange places, often in pain and full of anxiety.

Catholic teaching on death and care of the sick and dying does not say that life is unimportant or that medicine should not try to heal or save lives. Rather, it gives perspective to the meaning of health and death and their places in our lives. Callahan's position on premature death—that it should generally be avoided, but acceptable when the quality of life is gone or when further efforts to keep someone alive distorts the process of dying—is compatible with Catholic teaching on extraordinary and ordinary care.

The critical state of dying in America is a warning to all concerned about the common good to become advocates of broader reform of the way we distribute health care. The Catholic vision of death and care for the dying would want us to take the emphasis off expensive treatments for a few and place the emphasis on better services for all who need them.

Integrating Market Mechanisms

Catholic social thought supports the view that government is one of the best entities for protecting human dignity and promoting the common good. Justice requires accessible and affordable health care for all people. If we must use market mechanisms, then government must play a major role in the regulation and control of the activities of the market, in order to ensure that those mechanisms meet the requirements of justice. Which specific mechanisms could be used and still meet our requirements of justice? In order to answer this question, I will reexamine the widely used market mechanisms discussed in chapter 3.

Private insurance is so ingrained in American health care, I doubt we will see its demise very soon. It will most likely remain a primary mechanism in the funding of health care. The major problem with private insurance is many people do not have access to it, for several reasons. They do not have employer-provided insurance and cannot afford to pay for individual insurance. Or they are in high-risk health category and cannot get coverage. Private insurance must be made affordable and accessible to everyone.

Good federal public policy would require that all U.S. residents have health care coverage. This is the only way to guarantee universal coverage. Keeping in mind the principle of subsidiarity, some of the oversight can be delegated to the states because they are smaller entities and can help achieve a proper balance between reliance on small social units and on the federal government to meet the political, economic, and social obligations required of justice. Still, in order to maintain consistency and equity, the federal government should provide most of the oversight of the plan. This would mean that government must be able to monitor insurers so that monopolies do not emerge. Government can also provide economic incentives to encourage insurance companies to create affordable plans. It can oversee the organization of some type of insurance marketplace, such as the one proposed in the Massachusetts plan, which offers premium subsidies for low-income people who do not qualify for Medicaid, for small businesses to help cover their employees, and for individuals who are in high–health risk categories. The costs of such a system should be paid for by tax dollars because good health care benefits the good of the entire community.

Managed care has been under fire for years. John C. Robinson once described HMOs as "an economic success and a political failure."[96] People in the United States simply do not like having restrictions placed on their ability to choose whatever kind of medical care they want. However, it was exactly by restricting patients' and physicians' choices that managed care was able to keep costs down. The political and consumer backlash to these restrictions was so severe that lawsuits and legislation forced managed care to give up many of its cost-reducing policies, which eventually led to a failure to keep costs down. Still, managed care is excellent at providing integrative care. The inability to maintain cost-containing policies reflects more on the underlying values that drive our health care system, such as an undying love for individual desire and choice, than on poor economic planning.

User fees, copayments, and deductibles can help finance the system when, and only when, they do not interfere with accessibility to that system. Certainly, one could argue that any added cost will always influence an individual's decision whether to seek care. Still, there is no perfect system.

It is possible to take certain precautions to reduce the restrictive effect of fees so they meet the requirements of justice. One method for doing so is restricting the use of user fees, copayments, and deductibles for those considered low income or who have chronic illnesses. For example, in Belgium people who are considered low income are eligible to receive exemptions from health care cost sharing.[97] In Austria low-income people do not have to pay user fees for pharmaceuticals.[98] In France people who have any one of thirty diseases considered serious or chronic are exempt from user fees.[99] Under the Massachusetts plan, people at or below the poverty level do not have to pay deductibles. By providing for the waiver of copayments and deductibles for the poor and chronically ill, these market mechanisms can be used without impeding universal coverage and can therefore still make a financial contribution to the health care system.

Physician incentives have no place in a just health care system. Capitation, bonuses, and withholds merely put undue pressure on physicians to act as financial planners, instead of healers. There is little evidence to show that these mechanisms control costs, anyway. Most importantly, physician incentives erode public confidence in the medical profession. Trust is an essential ingredient for a just health care system. Even if physician incentives do not actually affect patient care, there is the perception that they do. This fact alone makes the case against their use.

Health accounts are available only to people with large disposable incomes. They do little to contain costs, improve efficiency, or improve access to health care. Therefore, they have minimal value in a just health care system.

Rationing Health Care

Although market mechanisms help fund health care, an equitable and sustainable health care system will not exist without rationing. Also known as supply-side controls, rationing is intended to control the production and distribution of health care products, rather than their consumption. Callahan correctly points out that we already ration health care. He refers to it as "soft rationing" because it is not legislated rationing. Instead, soft rationing occurs through practices that limit certain people's, particularly the poor's, access to health care. A just health care system cannot use soft rationing, because it discriminates against the poor and marginalized.

Rationing is a very controversial and unpopular topic in the United States, yet it must be addressed. There is not a significant amount of literature in Catholic thought on the rationing of health care. However, the Catholic Health Association (CHA) has put together one of the more comprehensive theological positions on this subject. In May 1990 the CHA appointed a working group on health care rationing to create criteria for evaluating methods. *With Justice for All? The Ethics of Health Care Rationing* was adopted by the CHA's Board of Trustees in February 1991. At the beginning of the document, the CHA states that "no society can afford to provide every healthcare service of potential benefits to everyone. Moreover, every society has important goals in addition to healthcare."[100] The CHA goes on to define rationing as "the withholding of potentially beneficial healthcare services because policies and practices establish limits on the resources available for healthcare."[101]

Acknowledging that the rationing of health care raises serious ethical questions, the CHA argues that, from the standpoint of Catholic social thought, the following eight ethical criteria can provide standards by which the use of rationing can be measured. First, the need for rationing must be demonstrable. There must still be a shortage in health care resources that remains even after all efforts have been made to eliminate waste, administrative costs, and excessive profit.[102] Second, health care rationing must promote the common good. Noting that health care is a social good that belongs to all, the CHA argues that there must be a balance between individual interests and the interests of local, state, and national communities, in order to serve the common good.[103] Third, a basic level of health care must be made available to everyone. CHA defines a basic level of health care as one that is "comprehensive to promote good health, to provide appropriate treatment for persons with disease and disability, and to care for persons who are chronically ill or dying."[104] The federal government should be responsible for guaranteeing that the health care financing mechanism is based on equity and a progressive taxation formula.[105]

The fourth criterion is that rationing must apply to everyone. The CHA is concerned because

> those most likely to construct and implement government rationing systems are not poor. Thus, unless this criterion is satisfied, those most likely to be denied healthcare will be those already most in need in society, whereas those who withhold this healthcare will be the relatively affluent.[106]

Because vital issues concerning life, death, and the quality of life are influenced by rationing, the fifth criterion calls for the policies governing rationing to be the result of a process that is open to participation by everyone. Sixth, the CHA gives an ethical priority to the unmet needs of the poor and uninsured, so "any government rationing proposal should be evaluated from their perspective and according to how it affects their lives."[107] Seventh, any rationing must be based on human dignity and therefore be free from "any wrongful discrimination based on age, gender, race, religion, national origin, education, place of residency, sexual orientation, ability to pay, or presumed social worth."[108] Finally, the CHA demands that the social and economic effects of any rationing must be closely monitored by government.[109]

Although the CHA's criteria are rather broad and do not offer any major details for implementing a rationing plan, they do provide a solid foundation upon which to think about rationing. Though Americans are especially adverse to the possibility of rationing, health care economist Thomas Rice argues, supply-side controls are very successful at cost containment. Commonly used supply-side controls in other developed countries with universal health care are the diffusion of medical technology, limits on hospital beds and physicians, and global budget controls.[110] Although such controls can result in limits on technology and waiting lists for certain health care services, Rice concludes that supply-side controls are a very effective way of containing costs while providing universal coverage.[111]

Hence, some type of health care rationing is necessary in order to guarantee the sustainability of a universal health care system. How can one make a winning case for rationing in the United States, with its severe distaste for the concept? If certain underlying values are changed, then the areas where health care can be rationed will become more obvious, and rationing may be easier to attain. For example, if good health is viewed merely as a means to achieve self-development, instead of a goal in and of itself, then it will be much easier to recognize that there are many other societal goods, that they are all required for self-development, and that they must all compete for support on an even playing field. Health care viewed in this light will be much easier to ration.

Conclusion: Can a Health Care Market Be Moral?

In the end we must reconsider health care. We must reexamine its place in our lives, how it is to define us, and how we are to respond to it. So often in life we are called to ask in whom and in what we are to believe. Catholic social thought answers that we are to believe in a loving Trinitarian God, whom we are to imitate by doing justice, which requires much of us. When it comes to health care, the most fundamental requirement is that some basic level of health care must be accessible to all. If such a system of health care is to exist and is to be able to provide enough minimal care so that humans are given a chance to develop fully, that system must have adequate financing to ensure its survival. When unchecked, market mechanisms in and of themselves challenge justice. They discriminate against the poor and disadvantaged of our society. They promote selfish and individualistic values. They often demoralize and commodify people.

Yet, some market mechanisms, such as private insurance, the integrative aspects of managed care, and user fees, copayments, and deductibles can be tamed so that they can provide much-needed financing to a health care system. Government can monitor them so they do not become leviathans. Their use can be restricted so that their effects on the poor and disadvantaged are minimal.

Still, if used alone, even with government oversight, market mechanisms are not the sole solutions to the vast problems facing health care today. The health care system is akin to a large jigsaw puzzle consisting of many facets. There are management and organizational facets that are very important. Market mechanisms can be good devices to shape these facets.

But these are merely a few pieces of the puzzle. In order to have a puzzle that truly fits together and portrays a universal and viable health care system, certain underlying values that drive the health care engine must be reconsidered. The value dimension approach of Daniel Callahan, combined with the vision of Catholic social thought, is an excellent source for doing just that. With its understanding of the meaning of life, health, illness and healing, suffering, and death, Catholic social thought provides substantive expression of the deeper values that affect the human condition and, thus, the health care system. Catholic social thought can accept certain market mechanisms for the funding and distribution of health care, provided they are integrated with the value dimension approach and interpreted within a Christian framework. If such a system is not developed, health care in the United States is going to see even greater disparities in coverage.

Notes

1. Catholic Health Association of the United States, *Continuing the Commitment*, 6–9.
2. Kaiser Family Foundation, *Key Facts*, 9.
3. Harrell and Carrasquillo, "Latino Disparity in Health Coverage," 1167.
4. Ibid.
5. Ibid.
6. Ibid.
7. Ibid.
8. Ibid.
9. Committee on the Consequences of Uninsurance, *Hidden Costs, Value Lost*, 65–66.
10. Ibid.
11. Ibid.
12. Ibid., 74.
13. Ibid., 75.
14. Ibid.
15. Ibid.
16. Lagnado, "Anatomy of a Hospital Bill," B1.
17. Ibid., B4.
18. Ibid.
19. Himmelstein et al., "Illness and Injury as Contributors to Bankruptcy," W5-69.
20. Ibid.
21. Ibid., W5-69.
22. Ibid., W5-70.
23. Ibid.
24. Ibid., W5-69–70.
25. Ibid., W5-71–72.
26. Committee on the Consequences of Uninsurance, *Hidden Costs, Value Lost*, 7.
27. Ibid., 69.

28. Curran, *Directions in Catholic Social Ethics*, 254.

29. Callahan, *What Kind of Life?* 58.

30. Curran, *Directions in Catholic Social Ethics*, 265.

31. Hussey et al., "How Does the Quality of Care Compare?"

32. Pellegrino, "Healing and Being Healed," 122.

33. Ibid.

34. Honnefelder, "Quality of Life and Human Dignity."

35. Callahan and Wasunna, *Medicine and the Market*, 73.

36. For an in-depth discussion of the increasing use of market mechanisms in developed countries, see ibid., ch.3.

37. Himes, *Responses to 101 Questions*, 55.

38. Callahan and Wasunna, *Medicine and the Market*, 43.

39. Zhang, "States Take a Look."

40. Angell, "Healthcare Plan Needs Dose."

41. Ibid.

42. Johnston and Turnbull, "Bold Insurance Experiment."

43. Ibid.

44. Zhang, "States Take a Look."

45. Lazarus, "Is Citywide Health Care Possible?"

46. United States Catholic Conference, *Catechism of the Catholic Church*, no. 1.

47. Paul VI, *Popularum progressio*, no. 15.

48. Ibid., no. 16.

49. McCormick, "Theology and Bioethics," 9.

50. Quoted in McCormick, *How Brave a New World?* 345–46.

51. Ibid., 346.

52. Ibid., 34–35.

53. Callahan, *What Kind of Life?* 37.

54. McCormick, *How Brave a New World?* 34.

55. Ibid.

56. Callahan, *What Price Better Health?* 87.

57. Ibid.

58. Pellegrino, "Healing and Being Healed," 115–16.

59. Ibid., 116.

60. Ibid.

61. Ibid., 117.

62. Ibid., 118.

63. Ibid.

64. Ibid.

65. Quoted in ibid., 119.

66. Ibid.

67. Aeschylus, *Three Greek Plays*, 170.

68. Quoted in De Schrijver, "From Theodicy to Anthropodicy," 108.

69. Frankl, *Man's Search for Meaning*, 11.

70. Ibid., 99.

71. Kreeft, *Making Sense out of Suffering*, 169.

72. Ibid., 170.

73. Ibid., 171.

74. Depoortere, *Different God*, 23–25.

75. Soelle, *Suffering*.

76. Texts are taken from the *Revised Standard Version of the Holy Bible*, Catholic ed.

77. Depoortere, *Different God*, 34.

78. Ibid., 36.

79. Ibid., 100.

80. Ibid., 101.

81. Ibid., 108.

82. United States Catholic Conference, *Catechism of the Catholic Church*, no. 1007.

83. Ibid., no. 1006.

84. Depoortere, *Different God*, 114.

85. Ibid., 117.

86. Wildes, "Ordinary and Extraordinary Means," 503–7.

87. Sacred Congregation, *Declaration on Euthanasia*, sec. IV.

88. Ibid.

89. Ibid.

90. United States Catholic Bishops, *Ethical and Religious Directives*, n. 58.

91. Shannon and Walter, "Implications of the Papal Allocution," 18.

92. Last Acts, *Means to a Better End*, 27.

93. Ibid., 34.

94. Ibid., 13.

95. Ibid., 21.

96. Robinson, "End of Managed Care," 2622.

97. Saltman and Figueras, *European Health Care Reform*.

98. Organization of Economic Cooperation and Development, "Reform of Health Care Systems."

99. Rodwin and Sander, "Health Care under French National Health."

100. Catholic Health Association of the United States, *With Justice for All?* 3.

101. Ibid., 6.

102. Ibid., 20.

103. Ibid., 21.

104. Ibid., 32.

105. Ibid., 34.

106. Ibid., 22.

107. Ibid., 23–24.

108. Ibid., 24.

109. Ibid., 25.

110. Rice, *Economics of Health Reconsidered*, 261.

111. Ibid., 256–62.

BIBLIOGRAPHY

Administration Board of the National Catholic Welfare Conference. *Our Bishops Speak*. Milwaukee: Bruce, 1952.

Aeschylus. *Three Greek Plays*. Translated by Edith Hamilton. New York: W. W. Norton, 1937.

Aetna Health Inc., fka Aetna U.S., Healthcare Inc., et al. v. Davila, 542 U.S. 200, 124 S. Ct. 2488, 159 L.Ed. 2d 319 (2004).

Angell, Marcia. "Healthcare Plan Needs Dose of Common Sense." *Boston Globe*, April 17, 2006, A4.

Aristotle. *Nicomachean Ethics*. Translated by Terence Irwin. 2nd ed. Indianapolis: Hackett, 1999.

Arrow, Kenneth J. "Uncertainty and the Welfare Economics of Medical Care." *American Economic Review* 53, no. 5 (1963): 941–73.

Augustine. *City of God*. Translated by Gerald G. Walsh, Demetrius B. Zema, Grace Monahan, and Daniel J. Honan. New York: Doubleday, 1958.

Baldwin, William. "Unsocializing Medicine." *Forbes* 169, no. 11 (2002): 24.

Bissonnette-Pitre, Lynne. "The Brief History of the CMA." Catholic Medical Association. www.cathmed.org/aboutthecma/ourhistory.htm (accessed November 11, 2006).

Bokenkotter, Thomas. *Church and Revolution: Catholics in the Struggle for Democracy and Social Justice*. New York: Image Books, 1998.

Bonino, José Míguez. *Doing Theology in a Revolutionary Situation*. Maryknoll, NY: Orbis Books, 1975.

Brown, E. Richard. "Public Policies to Extend Health Care Coverage." In *Changing the U.S. Health Care System: Key Issues in Health Services, Policy, and Management*, edited by Ronald M. Anderson, Thomas H. Rice, and Gerald F. Kominski, 31–57. San Francisco: Jossey-Bass, 2001.

Brown, Peter. *Augustine of Hippo*. Berkeley: University of California Press, 1967.

Cahill, Lisa Sowle. *Theological Bioethics: Participation, Justice, and Change*. Washington, D.C.: Georgetown University Press, 2005.

Cahill, Thomas. *Pope John XXIII*. New York: Penguin, 2002.

Callahan, Daniel. *False Hopes: Why America's Quest for Perfect Health Is a Recipe for Failure*. New York: Simon & Schuster, 1998.

———. "How Much Medical Progress Can We Afford? Equity and the Cost of Health Care." *Journal of Molecular Biology* 319 (2002): 885–90.

———. "Medical Technology, Innovation, and the Nature of Medical Progress." Paper presented at the Meeting on the Dissemination of Technological Innovation, Washington, D.C., January 12, 2003.

———. "Promises, Promises: Is Embryonic Stem-Cell Research Sound Public Policy?" *Commonweal* 132, no. 1 (2005): 12–14.

———. *Setting Limits: Medical Goals in an Aging Society.* Washington, D.C.: Georgetown University Press, 1995.

———. *The Troubled Dream of Life: In Search of a Peaceful Death.* Washington, D.C.: Georgetown University Press, 2000.

———. *What Kind of Life? The Limits of Medical Progress.* Washington, D.C.: Georgetown University Press, 1990.

———. *What Price Better Health? Hazards of the Research Imperative.* Berkeley, CA: University of California Press, 2003.

———, and Angela A. Wasunna. *Medicine and the Market: Equity v. Choice.* Baltimore: Johns Hopkins University Press, 2006.

Catholic Health Association of the United States. *Catholic Health Care in the United States.* St. Louis: Catholic Health Association of the United States, 2006.

———. *Continuing the Commitment: A Pathway to Health Care Reform.* St. Louis: Catholic Health Association of the United States, 2000.

———. "Health Care in America: A Reference Guide." St. Louis: Catholic Health Association of the United States, 2004.

———. "Ministry Engaged." St. Louis: Catholic Health Association of the United States, 2004.

———. *With Justice for All? The Ethics of Healthcare Rationing.* St. Louis: Catholic Health Association of the United States, 1991.

Catholic Medical Association. "Health Care in America: A Catholic Proposal for Renewal." *Linacre Quarterly* 72, no. 2 (2005): 92–122.

Centers for Disease Control and Prevention. *National Vital Statistics: Final Data for 2001.* Hyattsville, MD: Centers for Disease Control and Prevention, 2003.

Chadwick, Owen. *A History of the Popes, 1830–1914.* Oxford, England: Clarendon Press, 1998.

Christensen, Kate. "Ethically Important Distinctions among Managed Care Organizations." *Journal of Law, Medicine and Ethics* 23 (1995): 223–29.

Committee on the Consequences of Uninsurance of the Institute of Medicine. *Hidden Costs, Value Lost: Uninsurance in America.* Washington, D.C.: National Academies Press, 2003.

———. *A Shared Destiny: Community Effects of Uninsurance.* Washington, D.C.: National Academies Press, 2003.

Copleston, Frederick. *A History of Philosophy.* Vol. 8, *Modern Philosophy.* New York: Image Books, 1994.

Coppens, Charles. *Moral Principles and Medical Practices: The Basis of Medical Jurisprudence.* New York: Benziger, 1897.

Cornwell, John. *Hitler's Pope: The Secret History of Pius XII.* New York: Viking Press, 1999.

Curran, Charles. *Directions in Catholic Social Ethics.* Notre Dame, IN: University of Notre Dame Press, 1985.

———. *Issues in Sexual and Medical Ethics.* Notre Dame, IN: University of Notre Dame Press, 1978.

———. *Moral Theology: A Continuing Journey.* Notre Dame, IN: University of Notre Dame Press, 1982.

———. *Tensions in Moral Theology.* Notre Dame, IN: University of Notre Dame Press, 1988.

Depoortere, Kristiaan. *A Different God: A Christian View of Suffering.* Louvain Theological & Pastoral Monographs 17. Louvain, Belgium: Peeters Press, 1995.

De Schrijver, Georges. "From Theodicy to Anthropodicy: The Contemporary Acceptance of Nietzsche and the Problem of Suffering." In *God and Human Suffering,* edited by Jan Lambrecht and Raymond F. Collins, 95–119. Louvain, Belgium: Peeters Press, 1990.

Devettere, Raymond J. *Practical Decision Making in Health Care Ethics.* 2nd ed. Washington, D.C.: Georgetown University Press, 2000.

Dolan, Timothy M. "The Bishops in Council." *First Things* 152 (2005): 20–25.

Economist. "A Survey of the Human Genome." 356 (2000): 1–16.

Enthoven, Alain. "Consumer-Choice Health Plan (Part One)." *New England Journal of Medicine* 298, no. 12 (1978): 650–58.

———. "Consumer-Choice Health Plan (Part Two)." *New England Journal of Medicine* 298, no. 13 (1978): 709–20.

———. "Employment-Based Health Insurance Is Failing: Now What?" *Health Affairs* (Web Exclusive, May 28, 2003): W3 237–W3 249. Search "Enthoven + Employment" at www.healthaffairs.org (accessed November 11, 2006).

———. "The History and Principles of Managed Competition." *Health Affairs* 12 (Supplement 1993): 24–48. Search "Enthoven + History" at www.health affairs.org (accessed November 11, 2006).

———. "Market Forces and Efficient Health Care." *Health Affairs* 23, no. 2 (2004): 25–27.

———. *Theory and Practice of Managed Competition in Health Care Finance.* Amsterdam, The Netherlands: Elsevier Science, 1988.

———. "Why Not the Clinton Health Plan?" *Inquiry* 31 (1994): 129–35.

Folland, Sherman, Allen C. Goodman, and Miron Stano. *The Economics of Health and Health Care.* Upper Saddle River, NJ: Prentice-Hall, 1993.

Frankl, Viktor E. *Man's Search for Meaning*. Rev. ed. New York: Pocket Books, 1984.

Fraser, Barbara, and Paul Jeffrey. "A Call for Economic Change." *National Catholic Reporter* 40, no. 31 (June 4, 2004): 13–16.

———. "Poverty Cuts Children's Chances for a Future." *National Catholic Reporter* 41, no. 2 (October 29, 2004): 13–15.

Friedman, Milton. *Capitalism and Freedom*. Chicago: University of Chicago Press, 1962.

———. "Good Ends, Bad Means." In *The Catholic Challenge to the American Economy: Reflections on the U.S. Bishops' Pastoral Letter on Catholic Social Teaching and the U.S. Economy*, edited by Thomas M. Gannon, 99–106. New York: Macmillan, 1987.

———. "How to Cure Health Care." *Public Interest*, no. 142 (Winter 2001): 3–30.

Gabel, Jon, Gary Claxton, Erin Holve, Jeremy Pickreign, Heidi Whitmore, Kelley Dhont, Samantha Hawkins, and Diane Rowland. "Health Benefits in 2003: Premiums Reach Thirteen-Year High as Employers Adopt New Forms of Cost Sharing." *Health Affairs* 22, no. 5 (2003): 117–25.

Gaynor, Martin, and William B. Vogt. "What Does Economics Have to Say about Health Policy Anyway? A Comment and Correction on Evans and Rice." *Journal of Health Politics, Policy and Law* 22, no. 2 (1997): 475–508.

Goldstein, Amy. "For Patients' Rights, a Quiet Fadeaway." *Washington Post*, September 12. 2003, A4.

Groethuysen, Bernard. *The Bourgeois: Catholicism vs. Capitalism in Eighteenth-Century France*. New York: Holt, Rinehart & Winston, 1968.

Gutiérrez, Gustavo. *A Theology of Liberation*. Maryknoll, NY: Orbis Books, 1988.

Guyer, Bernard, Mary Anne Freedman, Donna M. Strobino, and Edward J. Sondik. "Annual Summary of Vital Statistics: Trends in the Health of Americans During the 20th Century." *Pediatrics* 106, no. 6 (2000): 1307–17.

Harrell, Joseph, and Olveen Carrasquillo. "The Latino Disparity in Health Coverage." *Journal of the American Medical Association* 289, no. 9 (2003): 1167.

Health Maintenance Organizations Act of 1973, United States Code, Title 42, ch. 6A, subch. XI, sec. 300e.

Herzlinger, Regina. "Consumer-Driven Health Insurance: What Works." In *Consumer-Driven Health Care: Implications for Providers, Payers, and Policymakers*, edited by Regina Herzlinger, 74–101. San Francisco: Jossey-Bass, 2004.

———. "Fear and Loathing of Defined Benefit Health Insurance." In *Consumer-Driven Health Care: Implications for Providers, Payers, and Policymakers*, edited by Regina Herzlinger, 3–27. San Francisco: Jossey-Bass, 2004.

———. "Health Care Productivity." In *Consumer-Driven Health Care: Implications for Providers, Payers, and Policymakers*, edited by Regina Herzlinger, 102–27. San Francisco: Jossey-Bass, 2004.

———. *Market-Driven Health Care: Who Wins, Who Loses in the Transformation of America's Largest Service Industry*. Paperback ed. Reading, MA: Addison-Wesley, 1997.

———. "More Market, Less Straightjacket." *Wall Street Journal*, January 22, 2004, A12.

———. "Prix-Fixe Rip-Off." *Wall Street Journal*, June 13, 2003, A16.

———. "Scare Stories, Opponents, and the Role of Government." In *Consumer-Driven Health Care: Implications for Providers, Payers, and Policymakers*, edited by Regina Herzlinger, 153–94. San Francisco: Jossey-Bass, 2004.

Herzlinger, Regina, and Ramin Parsa-Parsi. "Consumer-Driven Health Care in Switzerland." *Journal of the American Medical Association* 292, no. 10 (2004): 1213–20.

Himes, Kenneth. *Pacem in terris*. In *The Dictionary of Catholic Social Thought*, edited by Judith A. Dwyer, 696–706. Collegeville, MN: Liturgical Press, 1994.

———. *Responses to 101 Questions on Catholic Social Teaching*. New York: Paulist Press, 2001.

Himmelstein, David U., Elizabeth Warren, Deborah Thorne, and Steffie Woolhandler. "Marketwatch: Illness and Injury as Contributors to Bankruptcy." *Health Affairs* (Web Exclusive, February 2, 2005): W5-64–W5-73. Search "Himmelstein + Illness" at www.healthaffairs.org (accessed November 11, 2006).

Hollenbach, David. *Claims in Conflict*. New York: Paulist Press, 1979.

———. *The Common Good and Christian Ethics*. Cambridge, England: Cambridge University Press, 2002.

———. "The Common Good Revisited." *Theological Studies* 50 (1989): 70–94.

Honnefelder, Ludger. "Quality of Life and Human Dignity: Meaning and Limits of Prolongation of Life." In *Allocating Scarce Medical Resources: Roman Catholic Perspectives*, edited by H. Tristram Engelhardt, Jr., and Mark J. Cherry, 140–53. Washington, D.C.: Georgetown University Press, 2002.

Hunt, E. K., and Howard J. Sherman. *Economics: An Introduction to Traditional and Radical Views*. 4th ed. New York: Harper & Row, 1981.

Hussey, Peter S., Gerard F. Anderson, Robin Osborn, Colin Feek, Vivienne McLaughlin, John Miller, and Arnold Epstein. "How Does the Quality of Care Compare in Five Countries?" *Health Affairs* 23, no. 3 (2004): 89–99.

International Market Services. *I.M.S. Retail Drug Monitor*. 2005. Available from www.imshealth.com/.

International Theological Commission. "Communion and Stewardship: Human Persons Created in the Image of God." *Origins* 34, no. 15 (2004): 233–48.

John Paul II. "The Pope at Puebla." In *Puebla and Beyond*, edited by John Eagleson and Phillip Scharper, 47–83. Maryknoll, NY: Orbis Books, 1979.

———. *Centesimus annus.* In *Catholic Social Thought: The Documentary Heritage,* edited by David J. O'Brien and Thomas A. Shannon, 437–88. Maryknoll, NY: Orbis Books, 2000.

———. *Laborem exercens.* In *Catholic Social Thought: The Documentary Heritage,* edited by David J. O'Brien and Thomas A. Shannon, 350–92. Maryknoll, NY: Orbis Books, 2000.

———. *Redemptor hominis.* In *Proclaiming Justice and Peace: Documents from John XXIII–John Paul II,* edited by Michael Walsh and Brian Davies, 243–61. Mystic, CT: Twenty-Third Publications, 1984.

———. *Rich in Mercy:* Dives in misericordia. Washington, D.C.: United States Catholic Conference, 1981.

———. *Sollicitudo rei socialis.* In *Catholic Social Thought: The Documentary Heritage,* edited by David J. O'Brien and Thomas A. Shannon, 393–436. Maryknoll, NY: Orbis Books, 2000.

Johnston, Philip W., and Nancy C. Turnbull. "A Bold Insurance Experiment." *Boston Globe,* April 16, 2005, A6.

John XXIII. *Mater et magistra.* In *Catholic Social Thought: The Documentary Heritage,* edited by David J. O'Brien and Thomas A. Shannon, 82–128. Maryknoll, NY: Orbis Books, 2000.

———. *Pacem in terris.* In *Catholic Social Thought: The Documentary Heritage,* edited by David J. O'Brien and Thomas A. Shannon, 129–62. Maryknoll, NY: Orbis Books, 2000.

Jonsen, Albert R., and Stephen Toulmin. *The Abuse of Casuistry.* Berkeley: University of California Press, 1988.

Kaiser Commission on Medicaid and the Uninsured. *Health Care in America, 2004 Data Update.* Menlo Park, CA: Kaiser Family Foundation, 2005.

Kaiser Family Foundation/Health Research and Educational Trust. *Employee Health Benefits: 2003 Annual Survey.* Menlo Park, CA: Kaiser Family Foundation, 2003.

———. *Employee Health Benefits: 2004 Annual Survey.* Menlo Park, CA: Kaiser Family Foundation, 2004.

———. *Employer Health Benefits: 2003 Annual Survey.* Menlo Park, CA: Kaiser Family Foundation, 2003.

———. *For-Profit Health Care Comparisons: Trends and Issues.* Menlo Park, CA: Kaiser Family Foundation, 1998.

———. *Key Facts: Race, Ethnicity and Medical Care: June 2003 Update.* Menlo Park, CA: Kaiser Family Foundation, 2003.

———. *Trends and Indicators in the Changing Health Care Marketplace, 2002.* Menlo Park, CA: Kaiser Family Foundation, 2002.

———. *Trends and Indicators in the Changing Health Care Marketplace: 2004 Update.* Menlo Park, CA: Kaiser Family Foundation, 2004.

Keane, Philip S. *Catholicism and Health-Care Justice: Problems, Potential and Solutions.* New York: Paulist Press, 1999.

———. *Health Care Reform: A Catholic View.* New York: Paulist Press, 1993.

Kelly, David F. *Contemporary Catholic Health Care Ethics.* Washington, D.C.: Georgetown University Press, 2004.

———. *The Emergence of Roman Catholic Medical Ethics in North America.* New York: Edwin Mellen Press, 1979.

Kent, Peter C. *The Pope and the Duce: The International Impact of the Lateran Agreement.* New York: St. Martin's Press, 1981.

Kominski, Gerald F., and Glenn Melnick. "Managed Care and the Growth of Competition." In *Changing the U.S. Health Care System: Key Issues in Health Services, Policy, and Management,* edited by Ronald M. Anderson, Thomas H. Rice, and Gerald F. Kominski, 389–405. San Francisco: Jossey-Bass, 2001.

Kreeft, Peter. *Making Sense out of Suffering.* Ann Arbor, MI: Servant Books, 1986.

Lagnado, Lucette. "Anatomy of a Hospital Bill." *Wall Street Journal,* September 21, 2004, B1, B4.

Last Acts. *Means to a Better End: A Report on Dying in America Today.* Washington, D.C.: Last Acts, 2002.

Latin American Bishops Conference. "Medellín Documents: Justice." In *The Gospel of Peace and Justice: Catholic Social Teaching since Pope John,* edited by Joseph Gremillion, 445–54. Maryknoll, NY: Orbis Books, 1976.

———. "Medellín Documents: Peace." In *The Gospel of Peace and Justice: Catholic Social Teaching since Pope John,* edited by Joseph Gremillion, 455–64. Maryknoll, NY: Orbis Books, 1976.

Lazarus, David. "Is Citywide Health Care Possible?" *San Francisco Chronicle,* June 25, 2006, F1–F2.

Lieber, Ron. "The Health Savings Plan You Can't Get: Why Employers Are Slow to Try HSAs." *Wall Street Journal,* November 3, 2004, D1.

Leo XIII. *Humanum genus.* Rockford, IL: TAN Books, 1978.

———. *Quod apostolici muneris.* In *The Pope and the People: Select Letters and Addresses on Social Questions,* edited by Henry Parkinson, 28–40. London: Catholic Truth Society, 1914.

———. *Rerum novarum.* In *Catholic Social Thought: The Documentary Heritage,* edited by David J. O'Brien and Thomas A. Shannon, 12–39. Maryknoll, NY: Orbis Books, 2000.

Levinson, Jerome, and Juan de Onis. *The Alliance That Lost Its Way: A Critical Report on the Alliance for Progress.* Chicago: Quadrangle Books, 1970.

Locke, John. "Second Treatise on Civil Government." In *Social Contract: Essays by Locke, Hume, and Rousseau*, edited by Ernest Barker, 3–143. New York: Oxford University Press, 1947.

Managed Health Care Improvement Task Force. *Financial Incentives for Providers in Managed Care Plans Background Paper*. Oakland, CA: National Advisory Council on Professional and Organizational Ethics, 1999.

Marx, Karl. "Critique of the Gotha Program." In *The Marx-Engels Reader*, edited by Robert C. Tucker, 525–41. New York: W. W. Norton, 1978.

Massaro, Thomas. *Living Justice*. Lanham, MD: Sheed & Ward, 2000.

McCormick, Richard. *How Brave a New World? Dilemmas in Bioethics*. Garden City, NJ: Doubleday, 1980.

———. "Theology and Bioethics." *Hastings Center Report* 19 (1989): 5–10.

McFadden, Charles J. *Medical Ethics*. 2nd ed. Philadelphia: F. A. Davies, 1949.

McGinley, Laurie, and Sarah Lueck. "Behind Drug-Benefit Debate: How to Mix Medicare, Markets." *Wall Street Journal*, November 17, 2003, 1.

Mich, Marvin L. Krier. *Catholic Social Teaching and Movements*. Mystic, CT: Twenty-Third Publications, 1998.

Milio, Nancy. *Public Health in the Market: Facing Managed Care, Lean Government, and Health Disparities*. Ann Arbor: University of Michigan Press, 2000.

Morley, John F. *Diplomacy and the Jews during the Holocaust, 1939–1943*. New York: Ktav, 1980.

Muller, Jerry Z. *The Mind and the Market: Capitalism in Modern Thought*. New York: Alfred A. Knopf, 2002.

Murray, T. J. "Balancing Values, Funding and Americanization of Expectations in the Canadian Health System: An Historical Perspective." Paper presented at the Proceedings of the 37th International Congress on the History of Medicine, Galveston, TX, 2002.

National Conference of Catholic Bishops. *Ethical and Religious Directives for Catholic Health Care Services*. 4th ed. Washington, D.C.: United States Conference of Catholic Bishops, 2001.

———. "U.S. Bishops' Pastoral Letter on Health and Health Care." *Origins* 11, no. 25 (1981): 395–402.

Novak, Michael. "The Good Capitalist." *Christianity Today* (October 24, 1994): 29–31.

———. "Seven Theological Facets." In *Capitalism and Socialism: A Theological Inquiry*, edited by Michael Novak, 109–23. Washington, D.C.: Enterprise Institute for Public Policy Research, 1979.

———. *The Spirit of Democratic Capitalism*. New York: Simon and Schuster, 1982.

———. *Toward a Theology of the Corporation*. Washington, D.C.: Enterprise Institute for Public Policy Research, 1990.

Nozick, Robert. *Anarchy, State, and Utopia*. New York: Basic Books, 1974.

O'Brien, David J., and Thomas A. Shannon. "The Social Teaching of John Paul II." In *Catholic Social Thought: The Documentary Heritage*, edited by David J. O'Brien and Thomas A. Shannon, 347–50. Maryknoll, NY: Orbis Books, 2000.

Orentlicher, David. "Paying Physicians More to Do Less: Financial Incentives to Limit Care." *University of Richmond Law Review* 30 (1996): 155–72.

Organization of Economic Cooperation and Development. "The Reform of Health Care Systems: A Review of Seventeen OECD Countries." *Health Policy Studies* 5 (1999).

Paul VI. *Octogesima adveniens*. In *Catholic Social Thought: The Documentary Heritage*, edited by David J. O'Brien and Thomas A. Shannon, 265–86. Maryknoll, NY: Orbis Books, 2000.

———. *Popularum progressio*. In *Catholic Social Thought: The Documentary Heritage*, edited by David J. O'Brien and Thomas A. Shannon, 240–62. Maryknoll, NY: Orbis Books, 2000.

Pauly, Mark V. "Who Was That Straw Man Anyway? A Comment on Evans and Rice." *Journal of Health Politics, Policy and Law* 22, no. 2 (1997): 467–73.

———, Patricia Damon, Paul Feldstein, and John Hoff. "A Plan for 'Responsible National Health Insurance.'" *Health Affairs* 10, no. 1 (Spring 1991): 5–25. Search "Pauly + Plan" at www.healthaffairs.org (accessed November 11, 2006).

Pellegrino, Edmund D. "Healing and Being Healed: A Christian Perspective." In *Jewish and Catholic Bioethics: An Ecumenical Dialogue*, edited by Edmund D. Pellegrino and Alan I. Faden, 115–26. Washington, D.C.: Georgetown University Press, 1962.

Perez-Stable, E. J. "Managed Care Arrives in Latin America." *New England Journal of Medicine* 340, no. 14 (1999): 1110–12.

Peterson, Mark A. "Introduction: Health Care into the Next Century." In *Healthy Markets? The New Competition in Medical Care*, edited by Mark A. Peterson, 1–23. Durham, NC: Duke University Press, 1998.

Pius XI. *Quadragesimo anno*. In *Catholic Social Thought: The Documentary Heritage*, edited by David J. O'Brien and Thomas A. Shannon, 42–79. Maryknoll, NY: Orbis Books, 2000.

Pius XII. "Christmas Address, 1951." In *The Major Addresses of Pope Pius XII*. Vol. 2, edited by Vincent A. Yzermans, 149–73. St. Paul, MN: North Central, 1961.

———. "Pentecost Address, 1941." In *The Major Addresses of Pope Pius XII*. Vol. 1, edited by Vincent A. Yzermans, 26–36. St. Paul, MN: North Central, 1961.

Plato. *Plato's Republic*. Translated by G. M. A. Grube. Indianapolis: Hackett, 1974.

Plato. *The Republic of Plato*. Translated by Allan Bloom. 2nd ed. New York: Basic Books, 1968.

Rahner, Karl. "The Dignity and Freedom of Man." In *Theological Investigations*. Vol. 2, *Man and the Church*, 235–64. New York: Seabury, 1963.

Rawls, John. *A Theory of Justice*. Cambridge, MA: Belnap Press, 1971.

Revised Standard Version of the Holy Bible. Catholic ed. San Francisco: Ignatius Press, 1966.

Rhodes, Anthony. *The Vatican in the Age of the Dictators, 1922–1945*. New York: Holt, Rinehart and Winston, 1974.

Rice, Thomas H. *The Economics of Health Reconsidered*. 2nd ed. Chicago: Health Administration Press, 2003.

Robinson, James C. "The End of Managed Care." *Journal of the American Medical Association* 285, no. 20 (2001): 2622.

Rodwin, V. G., and S. Sander. "Health Care under French National Health Insurance." *Health Affairs* 12, no. 3 (1993): 111–31.

Rothstein, William G. "Pharmaceuticals and Public Policy in America: A History." In *Readings in American Health Care*, edited by William G. Rothstein, 375–91. Madison: University of Wisconsin Press, 1995.

Ryan, John A. *Distributive Justice*. New York: Macmillan, 1916.

———. *A Living Wage: Its Ethical and Economic Aspects*. New York: Macmillan, 1906.

Sacred Congregation for the Doctrine of the Faith. *Declaration on Euthanasia*. Boston: Pauline Books & Media, 1980.

Sacred Congregation for the Doctrine of the Faith. "Declaration on Euthanasia." *Origins* 10, no. 3 (1980): 155–56.

Saltman, Richard B., and Josep Figueras. *European Health Care Reform: Analysis of Current Strategies*. European Series 72. Copenhagen: WHO Regional Publications, 1997.

Second Vatican Council. *Gaudium et spes*. In *Catholic Social Thought: The Documentary Heritage*, edited by David J. O'Brien and Thomas A. Shannon, 166–237. Maryknoll, NY: Orbis Books, 2000.

Segundo, Juan Luis. *The Liberation of Theology*. Maryknoll, NY: Orbis Books, 1976.

Sen, Amartya. *Choice, Welfare, and Measurement*. Oxford, England: Basil Blackwell, 1982.

Shannon, Thomas A., and James J. Walter. "Implications of the Papal Allocution on Feeding Tubes." *Hastings Center Report* 34, no. 4 (2004): 18–20.

Sherman, Mark. "Health Care Spending Hits Record $1.7 Trillion, up 9.3 Percent in a Year." *San Francisco Chronicle*, January 8, 2004, A5.

Skinner, Wickham. "The Focused Factory." *Harvard Business Review* 52, no. 3 (May–June 1974): 113–22.

Smith, Adam. "*An Inquiry into the Nature and Causes of the Wealth of Nations*." In *Masterworks of Economics*. Vol. 1, *Mun, Turgot, Adam Smith, Malthus*, edited by Leonard Dalton Abbott, 58–179. New York: McGraw-Hill, 1973.

Smith, Christian. *The Emergence of Liberation Theology*. Chicago: University of Chicago Press, 1991.

Soelle, Dorothee. *Suffering*. Philadelphia: Fortress Press, 1975.

Starr, Paul. *The Social Transformation of American Medicine*. New York: Basic Books, 1982.

Synod of Bishops, 1971. "Justice in the World." In *Catholic Social Thought: The Documentary Heritage*, edited by David J. O'Brien and Thomas A. Shannon, 288–300. Maryknoll, NY: Orbis Press, 2000.

Taylor, Donald H. "What Price For-Profit Hospitals?" *Canadian Medical Association Journal* 166, no. 11 (2002): 1418–19.

Thomas Aquinas. *Summa Theologiae*. Vol. 2 in *Basic Writings of Saint Thomas Aquinas*, edited by Anton C. Pegis. Indianapolis: Hackett, 1997.

———. *Treatise on the Virtues*. Translated by John A. Oesterle. Notre Dame, IN: University of Notre Dame, 1966.

United States Catholic Conference. *Catechism of the Catholic Church*. New York: Doubleday, 1994.

U.S. Catholic Bishops, 1986. "Economic Justice for All." In *Catholic Social Thought: The Documentary Heritage*, edited by David J. O'Brien and Thomas A. Shannon, 572–680. Maryknoll, NY: Orbis Books, 2000.

U.S. Census Bureau. "Income, Poverty and Health Insurance Coverage in the U.S.: 2004." Washington, D.C.: U.S. Government Printing Office, 2006.

Vidler, Alec R. *The Church in an Age of Revolution*. London: Penguin Books, 1961.

Viner, Jacob. *Religious Thought and Economic Society*. Durham, NC: Duke University Press, 1978.

Wilcox, Sharon. "Promoting Private Health Insurance in Australia." *Health Affairs* 20, no. 3 (2001): 152–62.

Wildes, Kevin W. "Ordinary and Extraordinary Means and the Quality of Life." *Theological Studies* 57 (1996): 500–512.

Wolf, Charles. *Markets or Governments: Choosing between Imperfect Alternatives*. Cambridge, MA: MIT Press, 1993.

Yergin, Daniel, and Joseph Stanislaw. *The Commanding Heights*. New York: Simon & Schuster, 2002.

Zhang, Jane. "States Take a Look at Health Reform." *Wall Street Journal*, May 27–28, 2006, A4.

INDEX